Gaseous Detonations:

their nature, effects and control

Gaseous Detonations:
their nature, effects and control

MICHAEL A. NETTLETON

LONDON   NEW YORK

CHAPMAN AND HALL

First published in 1987 by
Chapman and Hall Ltd
11 New Fetter Lane, London EC4P 4EE
Published in the USA by
Chapman and Hall
29 West 35th Street, New York NY 10001

© 1987 Michael A. Nettleton

Printed in Great Britain by
J. W. Arrowsmith Ltd, Bristol

ISBN 0 412 27040 4

British Library Cataloguing in Publication Data

Nettleton, M. A.
  Gaseous detonations: their nature and control
  1. Gas dynamics   2. Explosions
  3. Shock waves
  I. Title
  533′.293   QC168.85.S45
  ISBN 0-412-27040-4

Library of Congress Cataloging in Publication Data

Nettleton, Michael A. (Michael Arthur), 1932–
  Gaseous detonations.

  Bibliography: p.
  Includes indexes.
  1. Explosions. 2. Shock waves. I. Title.
  QD516.N488 1986   620.8′6   86-13648
  ISBN 0-412-27040-4

Contents

Preface

My introduction to the fascinating phenomena associated with detonation waves came through appointments as an external fellow at the Department of Physics, University College of Wales, and at the Department of Mechanical Engineering, University of Leeds. Very special thanks for his accurate guidance through the large body of information on gaseous detonations are due to Professor D. H. Edwards of University College of Wales. Indeed, the onerous task of concisely enumerating the key features of unidimensional theories of detonations was undertaken by him, and Chapter 2 is based on his initial draft. When the text strays to the use of we, it is a deserved acknowledgement of his contribution. Again, I should like to thank Professor D. Bradley of Leeds University for his enthusiastic encouragement of my efforts at developing a model of the composition limits of detonability through a relationship between run-up distance and composition of the mixture. The text has been prepared in the context of these fellowships, and I am grateful to the Central Electricity Generating Board for its permission to accept these appointments.

I am most grateful to Academician Ya. B. Zel'dovich for his agreeing to spare some of his valuable time in commenting on the original draft and for writing a foreword. Since he always keeps me on my toes with his appropriate quotations from his encyclopaedic knowledge of the world's literature, it behoves me to reply πάντα ῥεῖ, οὐδὲν μένει (Heraclitus, 513 BC).*

It is also appropriate to acknowledge with sincere thanks the efforts of various illustrators who transformed my rough sketches into clear diagrams and those of a number of typists who patiently resigned themselves to dealing with numerous drafts of each chapter. Again, Dr G. O. Thomas, University College of Wales, kindly performed the C–J calculations given in Chapter 2.

A special vote of thanks is due to Mrs J. Finnigan, a colleague at Central

*All is flux, nothing is stationary.

Electricity Research Laboratories, who has painstakingly read both text and references. The contributions to the text from many discussions with co-workers in the field of detonations, too numerous to list individually, have been of inestimable value and are gratefully remembered; hopefully with complete accuracy.

Finally, an apology is owed to my daughters Naomi and Rebecca, for the times at which progress on the book was painfully slow, and my patience with them was not all that it should have been.

1985   Brockham
                                                        Betchworth
                                                        Surrey*

*As from 1988   Department of Mechanical Engineering
                 University of Queensland
                 St Lucia
                 Queensland
                 Australia 4067

Foreword

The idea of detonation came into being after disastrous explosions in coal mines more than a hundred years ago. The previous study of combustion concerned the slow process. The safety-grid-protected lamp of Davy and 'The story of a candle' by Faraday were the milestones of this line of investigation.

At first glance it was quite puzzling, how the slow subsonic combustion could produce strong mechanical effects. The understanding came after the laboratory experiments by the French investigators discovering the detonation of combustible mixtures in glass tubes.

Another source of our knowledge and interest in detonation came from pure theory. It is well known that the famous mathematician, Riemann, obtained the shock waves in inert media literally on the tip of his pen. He has shown that the movement of compressible gas leads to the formation of breaks with abrupt rise of pressure, density and temperature – even if the initial conditions were absolutely smooth. The contemporary reader would point to the nonlinearity of gasdynamic equations; he would call Riemann the ancestor of the modern catastrophe theory. The exact thermodynamics of the shock waves were found by Hugoniot. The generalization to chemically active media was not difficult and so the detonation theory of Chapman and Jouguet was born with the birth of the 20th century.

A puzzling point remained. The shock wave amplitude was dependent on the external causes of the shock. The detonation is a self-sustained process. Its properties must depend solely on the energy, density and other characteristics of the initial mixture. But formally the equations of Chapman and Jouguet were consistent with a set of final states. The authors had to put forward a new principle (minimal velocity or minimal entropy) in order to choose one point of the set. The principle worked well and in good agreement with the experiment. Still it had no firm theoretical foundation for forty years. It was Zeldovich (1940), Doring (1942) and von Neumann (1943) who independently found the underlying idea of combustion initiated by the shock wave going ahead of the chemical reaction zone.

But even these works were not the end of the story. The mining industry used high explosives. The detonation products with density more than twice that of water are not ideal gases. The eminent theoretician, Landau, together with Stanyukovich, has given an adequate description of the thermodynamics for this case. It opened the experimental study of dynamical megabar pressures. The money spent on Nobel prizes comes mainly from the solid explosives industry.

The further development of gas detonation has shown a complicated structure. The idealized Zeldovich-Doring-Neumann picture turned out to be unstable in the realistic case of chemical reactions which are strongly temperature dependent. An exact theory of detonation still does not exist!

A very important topic is the formation of detonation waves out of slow combustion. The landmark here was Shchelkin's experiment – the magic influence of a spiral turbilizing the gas motion before the flame. The role of the internal instability of the plane slow flame (Landau, Darrieux) is still not clear.

The purpose of the preceding short historical sketch ('all detonation in a nutshell') is to give the reader the impression of how complicated and many-faced is the subject of detonation. It shows also the very difficult task approached by the author – M. Nettleton. I do not think it is possible to make a uniform coverage of all the field, but the author has chosen a very important side of the problem. The main theme is the safety problems in handling combustible gas or dust mixtures with air or oxygen. Important exceptions are acetylene and ozone, which can detonate even in pure gas form, without air or combustibles mixed in.

The importance of the subject is obvious. Explosions and especially detonation in chemical industry lead to great life and economic losses. But the complexity of the problem is immense simply because catastrophes are treated by dealing with the unpredicted, situations not expected by the constructors. In these ill-defined situations general knowledge plus common sense are more useful than complicated mathematical theories and calculations.

I find the presentation by the author to be in accord with the goal. The book consists of nine chapters. After the introductory one Chapters 2 and 3 deal with the idealized and the real structure of the detonation wave.

The exposition is clear. An engineer or a student in technical sciences will use it without trouble and without the necessity of using other literature.

As a wish for the second edition, I would mention the question of losses. The losses of energy and impulse, as well as losses due to incomplete chemical reaction, are important. They lead to a decrease of detonation velocity and shock pressure as compared with the ideal thermodynamic calculation. Finally if the losses are greater than some definite value, they lead to the quenching of detonation. The theory of losses is made for a one-dimensional case only. Therefore it is not easy to give immediate answers to practical questions. Still it is important in principle.

The second topic which should be treated in greater detail is the question of intermediate regimes. In a pipe with rough walls (Shchelkin spiral) one can imagine the shock ignition when the shock wave is reflected by the spiral. But the bulk of the gas could be burned by a turbulent deflagration propagating from the walls to the centre of the tube. In connection with the overall picture pressures higher than Chapman–Jouguet are predicted.

The author points out on many occasions that mixtures near the limit are in some cases more dangerous than the stoichiometric ones. In this connection the experimental data of Zeldovich and Kogarko (Doklady Acad. Sci., USSR (1948) **63**, 553) should be mentioned.

In the next chapters, 4 and 5, the limits of detonation and its initiation are discussed. An approximate criterion for hydrocarbon mixture is given, based on experiment, with a sober comment on its universality. The importance of turbulence and hydrodynamical factors is well stressed. A special chapter contains complicated geometrical situations.

Very important is the warning of the author about cascade processes – first compression of the gas and then explosion or detonation of already compressed gas. As a maximum a 160:1 rise of pressure is quoted as possible compared with 20:1 in Chapman–Jouguet point.

Unusual, but very important for the engineer, are the last Chapters, 7, 8 and 9, about the stress and damage done by detonation, about detonation prevention and about the difficulties and pitfalls of the problem. The possible role of electrostatic charge and electric discharge is pointed out, and the last chapter made me remember the motto of the great physicist Niels Bohr 'The specialist is the man who knows what errors can be made in his field of knowledge'.

Extremely valuable is the literature – c. 400 references with the names of papers. Quite naturally I have the impression that the Russian literature on the subject should be represented stronger. There are about 30 references to Russian papers, most of them translated. I would easily double this number – but I am not sure if it would be fair, perhaps colleagues from other countries could do the same.

To end my foreword: to some extent it is question of age, not of nationality. For the younger researcher Riemann, Chapman, Jouguet, Zeldovich, Doring, von Neumann, Shchelkin are all in the same group of 'old staff' but for me, Shchelkin for example is an intimate friend whose early death I am still mourning.

The author of a book is always in danger of writing 'nothing about everything' – when broadening the subject, or of writing 'everything about nothing' – when giving more and more precision and details about one narrow question. It seems to me that Nettleton has found the sound middle way. He himself is a very active worker. The 30 references to his own works are proof of it. He has written a concise and useful book which can be recommended to all involved in detonation and safety.

Academician, Acad. Sci. USSR
Foreign Member of the Royal Society

Ya. B. Zeldovich

1

Introduction

1.1 General remarks

The increasing size and complexity of plant processing exothermically-reacting chemicals has highlighted the dangers associated with the possible formation of a detonation, both within the plant and for flammable chemicals, within a vapour cloud produced by an accidental spillage or leakage. Historical surveys of the explosion of vapour clouds [1] are particularly illustrative. The designer of such plant, containing potentially detonable gases, aerosols or clouds of dust, in the event of an excursion from normal conditions of operation, faces severe difficulties in obtaining appropriate data to safeguard the plant and its surrounds against the effects of a detonation wave. Thus, available information on composition limits and pressure limits of detonable media, on the intensity, on the distribution and on the duration of internal stresses is sparse and what is available is scattered throughout the literature. Part of the problem arises from the lack of a comprehensive theory describing the multi-dimensional nature of detonation fronts, the effects of which are most marked in the marginally-detonable media most likely to be encountered in fault conditions. This has resulted in the extended existence of oversimplified unidimensional theories of detonation fronts and their application to situations in which they can produce misleading results. However, the designer faces further ambiguities. In plant other than a spherical vessel at the centre of which a detonation is directly initiated, the interactions of the expansion and compression waves produced during the formation of the front, with changes in the shape of the confinement and the subsequent mutual interactions of the resultant waves are complex and have received little attention. Again, until recently there has been little information on equally complex processes involved as a steadily propagating detonation front interacts with a change in shape of the confining walls. It is worth noting that most of these problems are also encountered in assessing the effects of a potential detonation of a cloud of vapour on structures within the cloud itself. Indeed, the curvature of such a front, which will result in an extended interaction over a planar surface from which it reflects, arguably results in an even more complex problem. Only when the wave has refracted at the cloud–air interface and travelled for some distance into the surrounding atmosphere does its pressure profile assume the well-characterized N-shape of a blast front [2].

Whilst there have been a number of books devoted solely to the subject of gaseous detonations [3–7], significant sections in texts on both combustion [8, 9] and shock waves [10, 11] dealing with the subject, contributions in monographs on hazards in industrial processes [12, 13] and numerous reviews of advances in our understanding [14–17], none have addressed the needs of the designers of chemical plants, covering media in which detonations are likely to occur, their causes, effects and methods of control and mitigation of the effects. Only the review by Munday [18] has been written from an engineering standpoint. However, this only covers readily detonable media and assessment of damage. Furthermore, the latter relies on an oversimplistic treatment of a unidimensional detonation front which, as will be shown, can lead to dangerous underestimates of local internal stresses. The lack of an engineering approach to the subject is somewhat surprising in view of the pioneering studies in the United Kingdom by Dixon [19], prompted by a disastrous explosion in a 1 m diameter gas main in London in 1880. Dixon's studies included a number of observations on features of great practical importance; for instance, he reported on the generation of internal pressures in excess of those produced by a steady front at positions close to the origin of the front, on the effects of a bend on the local pressures generated by a detonation and on the processes involved in the reflection of two detonation fronts colliding head-on. The use of increasingly sophisticated experimental techniques to monitor these and related problems, described in Section 1.4, has resulted in significant advances in our understanding of the mechanisms involved. However, it would be idle to claim a complete appreciation of these and it is instructive to consider the reasons for this situation. Probably the most important cause is the relative success of the use of unidimensional models of detonation fronts in describing their global properties in media well removed from their detonation limits. Unidimensional models are described qualitatively in Section 1.3 and a full account is given in Chapter 2.

1.2 Definitions of commonly-used terms

Workers from a wide range of disciplines share an interest in the properties of gaseous detonations, so that it appears advisable at this stage to introduce some important terms widely used in the literature. Broadly, they can be divided into two categories: those describing aspects of fluid dynamics and those dealing with the chemistry of the process. Of all the terms, a *gaseous detonation* is undoubtedly the most difficult to define in a concise but precise fashion. Chapters 2 and 3, describing the original concept of steady and unidimensional waves and the experimental evidence clearly demonstrating their non-steady multidimensional nature respectively, make this point at some length. A helpful overall starting-point is to regard a detonation wave as a shock front which is supported by the energy released in one or more reaction zones in the flow behind it. As such the velocity of the leading front varies across its periphery and the velocities of the reaction zones are unsteady. Only the average properties of the leading front and the associated flow can be described from a consideration of the energy released in the reaction zones. Finally, the separation between reaction zones and the leading wave varies widely, depending on whether the detonation is travelling

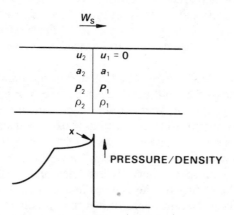

Figure 1.1 Flow conditions for a planar shock front, with x the relaxation zone in which vibrational modes reach equilibrium (von Neumann spike in detonations).

in a medium close to its limits of detonability or in a readily-detonable mixture and on whether it is a gaseous or two-phase medium. In contrast, a *deflagration wave* is used to describe all stages of flame development from propagation at the normal laminar burning velocity to the flame–shock complex prior to the completion of the coupling between reaction zones and the shock.

A *shock* is a wave front, the leading edge of which is only a few free molecular paths thick and across which pressure and density of the medium sharply increase (Fig. 1.1). The initial increase in energy is in the translational and rotational modes of the medium; the vibrational mode only achieves equilibrium at a later stage. The velocity of the front, W_s, is constant and is usually defined in non-dimensional terms as a Mach number $M_s = W_s/a_1$, where a_1 is the velocity of sound ahead of the front and $M_s > 1$. In contrast, a shock the velocity of which falls with distance to approach a Mach number of unity is defined as a blast wave. Useful parameters in assessing the effect of shocks and blasts on structures are *shock strength* and *overpressure*. The shock strength z is the ratio of pressure behind the front, p_2, to that ahead of it, p_1: $z = p_2/p_1$ and the overpressure $\Delta p = (p_2 - p_1)/p_1$. A particularly useful and commonly occurring abbreviation used to describe the gradients in gas velocity and sound speed behind curved shocks and those changing strength as they travel through a medium is *flow-field*. Obviously, from the definition above of a blast wave, gas velocities and sound speeds immediately behind the front decrease with distance travelled.

When confined detonations are produced by a flame accelerating through the mixture, a shock front and associated reaction zone (which travels back into the products of the initial flame) is commonly formed at the point of detonation. This is the so-called *retonation wave*, the properties of which have not been systematically studied. However, the leading front is a strong shock wave with $p_2/p_1 \leq 10$ and up to one-third of the heat of reaction can be released in the accompanying reaction zone, as the products tend to reach their equilibrium concentrations at the enhanced pressures and temperatures behind the front.

Turning now to chemical aspects of detonations, *stoichiometry*, ϕ, refers to the ratio of fuel to oxidant in the unreacted medium. For mixtures of hydrocarbons with oxygen or air, a stoichiometric mixture is conventionally one which is precisely composed to form carbon dioxide and steam as products. The convention is somewhat anomalous since the immediate products in the reaction zones include carbon monoxide, hydrogen, free radicals such as hydroxyl and atomic species such as hydrogen and oxygen, the relative concentrations depending on the composition of the unreacted medium. Mixtures with lower concentrations of fuel than is contained in a stoichiometric mixture are termed *fuel-lean* or *lean* and those with higher concentrations are denoted as *rich* mixtures. Obviously the definition of stoichiometry is even more arbitrary for oxidants such as the higher oxides of nitrogen, which are not completely converted to nitrogen, but a mixture of nitrogen and its lower oxides. Of crucial import to confined detonations originating from an accelerating flame is the laminar burning velocity of the medium S_u which is the velocity at which a flame advances orthogonally into a quiescent mixture. *Turbulent burning velocities*, S_t, are almost invariably defined in terms of S_u. However, this can give rise to difficulties when considering the appropriate corrections to be applied to the flow velocities ahead of turbulent flames, when the dimensions of wrinkles in the front differ greatly. A further important variable governing the acceleration of flames is the *expansion ratio* ϵ, the ratio of the density of the unreacted medium to that of the products $\epsilon = \rho_u/\rho_p$. Finally, in the context of the distribution of reaction zones in the flow behind the leading wave, *ignition delays* (τ_{ig}) and *energies of activation*, E_a, are important parameters. The ignition delay is the time elapsed between shock compression and heating of the detonable medium and the onset of exothermic chemical reactions, generally associated with the recombination of radicals and atomic species. The recombination steps are preceded by a set of reactions leading up to a chain-branching step in which the reaction of one radical or atomic species with a molecular species results in the production of two active species e.g.

$$H^\bullet + O_2 \rightarrow HO^\bullet + O^\bullet$$

The exponential dependence of the rate of such reactions on the temperature of the medium is expressed in terms of an energy of activation, which is high for initiating steps such as dissociation, lower for the attack of radicals on molecular species and approaches zero for recombination steps.

1.3 Unidimensional models of detonations

Unidimensional models involve simple considerations of the coupling of the leading shock front, the velocity of which depends on the nature of the fuel and the composition of the detonable medium (but generally lies in the range 1.5 to 4.0 km s^{-1} ($4 \leq M \leq 8$)) and a reaction zone travelling behind it at the same velocity. The original model proposed independently by Chapman [20] and Jouguet [21], hereafter denoted the C–J model, incorporates an energy input term in the conventional Rankine–Hugoniot analysis. It is related to the velocity of the front, D_{C-J}, through the assumption that the composition of the products corresponds with equilibrium at the temperature and density in the flow behind it. The model is commonly used to produce reliable predictions of global velocities measured under conditions in which thermal and viscous losses are negligible. It indicates they differ for various fuels and they depend on the composition of the mixture, but gives no information on detonation limits. It is open to the obvious criticism that reaction rates are finite, so that the implicit assumption of energy addition at the plane of the leading shock is unjustifiable. Following objections of this kind, and considering the possible magnitude of thermal and viscous losses from the zone separating shock and the plane at which chemical equilibrium is reached, led to the development of the Zel'dovich [22], von Neumann [23], Doring [24] (ZND) model.

The original ZND model is based on the concept of the leading shock producing a flow of the requisite density and temperature to trigger exothermic reactions at a short distance (1–10 mm) behind the shock, depending on the losses in this region. Subsequent developments have resulted in an increasingly sophisticated model: thus, the gas treated by the leading shock is initially excited in only the translational and rotational modes, and the delay during which equilibrium with the vibrational modes is attained is one during which abnormally high pressures occur. At the temperatures and densities of the flow immediately behind a typical detonation front, an equilibrium distribution of thermal energy should be achieved in not more than a few microseconds. Thus, the von Neumann pressure spike is of short duration (Fig. 1.1). Again, expressions which more realistically represent ignition delays (τ_{ig}) for chain reactions, generally involved in detonations, have been introduced into the model in order to estimate the separation between the shock and reaction zone. These relate the time required for the onset of recombination reactions of the type

$$H^{\bullet} + OH^{\bullet} + M \rightarrow H_2O + M,$$

responsible for the major portion of energy released in Arrhenius form

$$\tau_{ig} = [F]^m [O_x]^n \exp (E_a/RT) \tag{1.1}$$

where $[F]$ and $[O_x]$ are the concentrations of fuel and oxidant respectively, E_a a global activation energy, R the gas constant and T the equilibrium temperature in the flow behind the leading front. The extension of the model offers the possibility of estimating composition limits of detonability for confined mixtures [25, 26]. Substituting experimental values of m, n and E_a in Equation 1.1 leads to estimates of $1 \leq \tau_{ig} \leq 10$ μs at the temperature and density of the flow behind a shock propagating at a velocity typical of a detonation wave. In turn, these times suggest that the separation of leading shock and reaction zone in gaseous mixtures is typically in the range 1–10 mm. By considering energy losses from a plug of gas of this range the attenuation in velocity due to viscous forces can be calculated and a limit defined by an arbitrary choice of decrement in velocity.

While one-dimensional models afford a convenient framework for discussing the properties of the front itself and can be further developed to indicate the mechanisms governing detonation limits, they fail to give any guidance on the complex interactions of detonations with confinement. In order to understand these interactions, the multi-dimensional nature of a detonation must be considered. The appreciation of the importance of the structure of the front has grown from the early discovery of 'spinning' fronts [27, 28]. Unfortunately, severe problems have been encountered in suitably combining a fluid dynamic analysis of the properties of the leading front with a comprehensive treatment of the chemical kinetics in the reaction zones, and have resulted in the development of theory lagging well behind the growth in experimental data on the structure of detonation fronts and its relationship with confinement. In the continued absence of more appropriate models, C–J and ZND models are widely used – for example, detonation velocities and their variation with the composition of the mixtures and temperature, pressure and density ratios across the leading front are almost invariably computed, with generally satisfactory accuracy, from readily-available programs [29–31] based on unidimensional models. Thus, a fuller appreciation of the implications of such models is necessary and a more formal description is given in Chapter 2.

1.4 Structure of a detonation wave

At this stage it is appropriate to include a brief description of the principal features of a real detonation wave and how far they depart from the idealized concepts of unidimensional theory. This is expanded in Chapter 4, in terms of the effects on local pressures produced by the interaction of a detonation with confining walls. Presently, it suffices to trace the growing body of evidence for the multi-dimensional nature of detonation waves through the historical development of increasingly sensitive monitoring techniques. In addition, the relationship of the rudimentary theoretical treatments of real detonation waves (which are in course of development) with unidimensional models is examined. The inclusion of readily-available data from unidimensional models (such as the C–J velocity) in treatments of structure emphasizes the importance of an appreciation of the earlier theories and draws attention to the potential pitfalls in an unwary approach to published data.

Early and compelling evidence for the non-steady and multi-dimensional nature of detonation came from records of the interactions of the fronts with deposits on the walls of the detonation tube. For instance, confirmation of 'spinning' detonation fronts in moist mixtures of carbon monoxide with

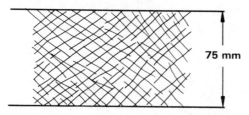

75 mm

Figure 1.2   Idealized sketch of smoked foil record of a detonation in a stoichiometric mixture of acetylene and oxygen at 110 torr.

oxygen was obtained from spiral tracks etched by the fronts in a silver deposit on the surface of glass tubes of circular cross-section. Further development of the technique led to the almost universal use of thin deposits of soot on the walls of the detonation tube or as a thin plate over which the front travels in studies of spherically-expanding fronts. A sketch of a typical soot track pattern from a confined detonation in a stoichiometric mixture of acetylene with oxygen is shown as Fig. 1.2. Systematic studies of the influence of the type of fuel, of composition and initial pressure of the mixture and of diluents on the dimensions of the cells making up the pattern have done much to classify the nature of detonation fronts. Thus, it was appreciated that the patterns implied a regular distribution of perturbations on the leading front and these were identified with triple-shock configurations, similar to those produced by planar shocks in non-reactive media diffracting on wedges of small angles of incline. A typical example is sketched in Fig. 1.3. The three shocks consist of the Mach stem, OM, the incident wave, IO and the reflected shock, OR (more commonly the transverse wave). The velocity of OM is increased by the process of diffraction, so that the pressure in the flow behind it is increased to the same level as that of the flow treated by both IO and OR. Mixture processed by the Mach stem only is separated from that processed by a combination of incident and reflected shocks by a contact surface (slipstream), OS.

Soot tracks are inscribed by the Mach stems of two sets of triple-shock configurations travelling orthogonally to each other. The triple points in each set collide with their neighbours and reflect; those closest to any confining wall reflect from it. Thus, the technique performs most satisfactorily for media in which detonation maintains a regular pattern. For mixtures close to the limits of detonability and for the majority of hydrocarbon fuels the patterns are highly irregular, so the vast majority of experimental studies of this kind have been carried out in mixtures close to stoichiometric composition, at initial

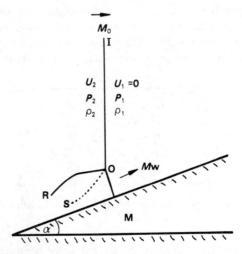

Figure 1.3   Mach reflection of a planar shock by a wedge angle α, with IO the incident wave, OM the Mach stem, OR the reflected wave (transverse front) and OS the contact surface (slipstream).

pressures below 1 bar and frequently with the mixtures heavily diluted by argon. Such measures enhance the reproducibility and legibility of the patterns.

Various high-speed photographic techniques have been used to confirm the multidimensionality of detonation fronts. For instance, in studies of the diffraction of detonation waves at an abrupt change in area an open-shutter camera technique has been used to produce photographic patterns equivalent to soot tracks [32]. They result from the intense luminosity of the triple points and the spatial resolution, provided by the velocity of the leading front. Schlieren methods, using short-duration background illumination to freeze the motion, can also be used to identify the structure associated with triple-point configurations in the flow. Figure 1.4 is a series of sketches of such records of a detonation in a stoichiometric oxyhydrogen mixture diffracting

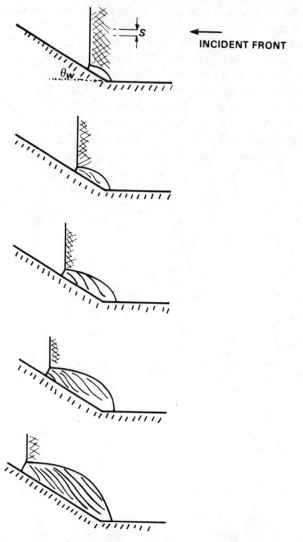

Figure 1.4 Diffraction of a detonation in $2H_2 + O_2 + Ar$ on wedge $\Theta_w = 30°$ [33] (5 μs intervals between successive records).

along a wedge of inclination 30°, and demonstrates clearly the changes in structure behind the incident front and Mach stem [33]. Interferographic systems, based (as are schlieren methods) on changes in gradients of refractive index across the various shocks have only been infrequently used, probably on account of their increased complexity. However, when they have been resorted to, they also illustrate the existence of one or more transverse fronts.

The lag between the onset of a detonation and its detection in metal pipelines may be reduced by monitoring the passage of a stress wave through the walls, since its velocity is some two to three times that of the detonation wave. Another technique which is suitable for pipeline bends, in which line-of-sight methods would fail, makes use of a wire stretched along the axis and modestly charged to about 10 V with respect to the walls [34]. Following the onset of a detonation the enhanced ionization results in an increase in voltage by a factor of five to ten in a resistor in series with the wire.

Streak schlieren is a particularly useful method for continuously monitoring the velocity of the leading front. Figure 1.5 is a sketch of a streak schlieren

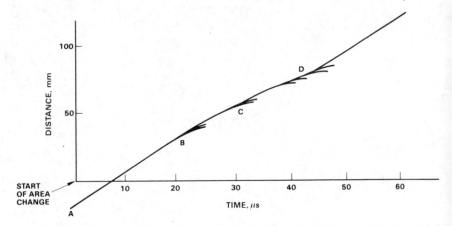

Figure 1.5   Sketch of a streak schlieren of decay and re-establishment of a detonation in a stoichiometric mixture of oxygen and acetylene travelling through an abrupt expansion in area [35].

record of the axial propagation of a detonation in a stoichiometric oxy-acetylene mixture through an abrupt change in area [35]. The constant velocity incident wave from A to B starts to fail between B and C and begins to re-establish itself between C and D to produce a constant velocity front from D onwards. A very sophisticated streak schlieren system, capable of resolving the features of a detonation with only one transverse front (spinning wave) is described in detail in Chapter 3.

Although the levels of ionization in the reaction zones of detonations [36] (electron density typically 10^{18} m^{-3}) are only an order of magnitude or so higher than the maximum levels in normal hydrocarbon flames and are much lower than those typical of the channel of an initiating spark [37] (10^{22} m^{-3}), they are sufficiently high for substantial reflection of microwave radiation. Thus, microwave interferometry, based on the difference in frequency between the radiation incident on and reflected from the front, is a particularly useful technique in that it minimizes any effect of the observation on the measured parameter. In addition, it can be used to record continuously the variations in velocity of dust suspensions where optical methods and smoked-foil records are ruled out by the presence of the particles. Typical interferograms, representing the success and failure to initiate a detonation in a suspension of coal dust in a mixture of oxygen and nitrogen contained in a tube from a C–J wave in a stoichiometric oxyacetylene mixture [38], are shown in Fig. 1.6. The initial portions of the interferograms represent the

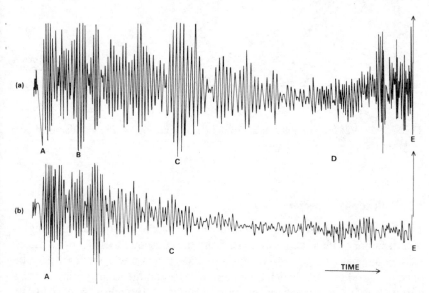

Figure 1.6 Microwave interferometry records of (a) accelerating coal dust flame and (b) attenuating blast front from an initiating oxyacetylene detonation [38].

decay of the detonation in an oxyacetylene mixture to a blast wave in air and in the suspension. Whilst the frequencies are similar in regions BC, the mixture with coal present results in much higher amplitudes of signal, presumably on account of the release of readily ionizable materials (such as sodium chloride) from the coal. The frequencies in the presence and absence of coal dust begin to differ appreciably at D, as the particles ignite in the flow behind the blast front. The record terminates as the leading front reaches the microwave aerial. Typical velocity versus distance plots from such interferograms for two mixture compositions $\lambda = 0.76$ and 1.2 are illustrated in Fig. 1.7. The oscillations in velocity at distances >1.5 m during the transition to a steady detonation front are mirrored in variations in pressure, emphasizing the dangers of local pressures greatly in excess of those anticipated during initiation [39–40].

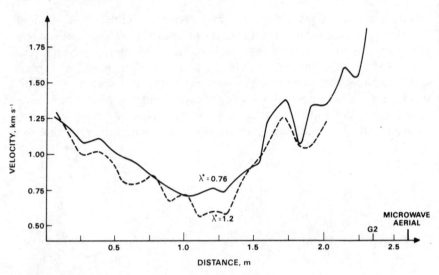

Figure 1.7 Velocity of ionization front in a suspension of 25 μm diameter coal particles [38]; ——— λ = 0.76, - - - λ = 1.2.

1.5 Philosophy of presentation

The flow-chart shown as Fig. 1.8 illustrates the probable sequence of thoughts of a designer of plant at possible risk from the consequences of a detonation. It is equally applicable to systems in which a detonable medium may be produced and to those which are potentially vulnerable to the possibility of a detonation in an unconfined cloud of vapour. Although at first sight the complete specification of the composition of the potentially detonable medium presents no problems, further examination makes it obvious that it is not the case. Consider the case of a plant built close to a shipping lane, on a port facility, or close to road and railways and assume its lifetime is some tens of years. In such a span the nature of flammable materials transported is likely to change markedly, for instance from present day cargoes of oil-based hydrocarbons to hydrogen and synthetic fuels in future. Thus, the consequences of a leak forming a vapour cloud and its subsequent possible detonation may require continual reassessment. Again, it is not unknown for plant manufacturing a particular product to be modified to produce an alternative product. Perhaps of even more concern, the occurrence of fault conditions on plant, for instance an excursion in temperature in the reaction vessel, might well result in a change in the principal product.

Having positively identified the fuel itself and the probable composition and pressure of the medium, there is the problem of identifying whether the medium is in fact capable of supporting a detonation. There are difficulties in presenting available data in a manner most appropriate to answering this question. We have decided that the most helpful way is to deal with the historical models of idealized detonations in Chapter 2 and indicate their shortcomings in Chapter 3, illustrating the experimental evidence for the multi-dimensional nature of detonations. This appears to be the most logical approach, in that variables such as the C–J velocity calculated from unidimensional models and its modifications to take account of the multi-dimensional nature of the wave are required, in order to answer questions on potential detonability. Whilst there is a voluminous literature on unidimensional detonations, we have tried to reduce references to a minimum, associated

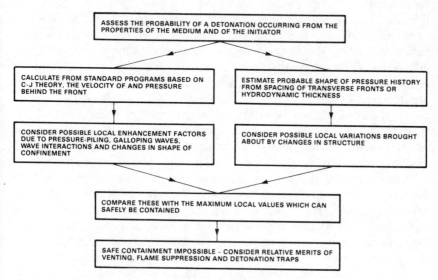

Figure 1.8   Designing for the possibility of a detonation.

with the aim of clarifying the aspects which are currently in use in descriptions of detonable medium. Having done so, it seems important to point out why the orderly and widely-applicable analyses presented are not universally applicable to assessments of the vulnerability of plant. Chapter 3 presents some of the experimental evidence for the multi-dimensional nature of detonations, emphasizing the possibility of the occurrence of pressures well in excess of those predicted by unidimensional theories [39, 40]. In many instances the multi-dimensionality of detonations is often most clearly demonstrated in their interactions with changes in confinement. However, Chapter 3 deals in the main with the important influence of composition and pressure of the mixture on the structure of the front, in the absence of any changes in the shape of confinement.

The idea that all self-decomposing fuels and mixtures of fuel and oxidant, together with the conditions of initial pressure and degree of confinement required for the formation of a detonation, have been identified is reassuring, but unfortunately erroneous. Frequently, identification of hazardous media is the result of an accident. Consequently, we have taken care to reference Chapter 4 on detonable media as exhaustively as possible. However, it is still necessary to include the caveat that many other media, especially at elevated temperatures and pressures, may support a detonation. Unfortunately, solutions to the C–J equations, indicating the existence of a front of the velocity typical of a detonation, occur for mixtures which are known to lie well outside the limits of detonability. Again, there has been too little work on unidimensional models which take into account losses from the front to have full confidence in their predictions of limits in a variety of media. Potentially the most reliable indicator for assessing detonability of a medium lies in a prediction of whether it is capable of sustaining at least one transverse wave behind a leading shock of approximately C–J velocity. There are grave difficulties in producing a theoretical treatment which combines a description of the fluid dynamics of the shock fronts and the complex chemical kinetics occurring in the reaction zones. Consequently, the development of a general model of complete dependability based on this yardstick is unlikely, so that it is advisable, in the event of a malfunction of plant, to test any medium for which experimental information is unavailable. The test should be carried out under the most extreme conditions of temperature and pressure possible.

For mixtures of fuel and oxidant, limits of detonability are frequently assessed in terms of flammability limits. Since limits of detonability are generally narrower than limits of flammability (with the possible exception of pure acetylene [41]), there is a case for basing conservative design on the latter. The consideration of detonations originating from accelerating flames [42] calls attention to the twin requirements of an appropriate medium and the existence of some ignition source for the indirect formation of a detonation. The energy required from an ignition source is much lower than the energy needed for the direct initiation of a detonation. Consequently, the probability of indirect initiation of a confined detonation is higher than that for direct initiation. Chapter 5 describes and compares both modes of initiation of a detonation in some detail. In particular, it contains a comprehensive review of energy requirements for both forms of initiation of confined and unconfined detonations, in order to assess the possibility of safety procedures based on the exclusion of sources of greater than a minimum level.

For confined detonations, there is a minimum length of pipeline (usually denoted the run-up distance) over which the flame must accelerate, first to form a shock in the medium ahead of it and subsequently for the transition to detonation. The possibilities of increasing the safety of plant by ensuring that lengths of pipelines nowhere exceed the run-up distances are obvious. A novel analysis of run-up distances is included in Chapter 5 and shown to afford tolerable predictions of these for the relatively few mixtures which have been studied experimentally. A bonus from this model is that when it is used to assess the effects of composition on run-up distances, the asymptotes to infinite run-up distances give lean and rich limits. On account of the wide potential utility of run-up distances, details of the effects of pressure, temperature and composition of the mixture and pipeline diameter on run-up distances are described in some detail. Chapter 5 concludes with a review of the dangers of anomalously high pressures being generated by detonations propagating into media which have been precompressed by compression waves, arising either from the initiator or from the structured nature of the front.

Should available data suggest that it is possible for a mixture within the limits of detonability to occur, and that it is impossible to exclude all initiating sources or to ensure that the lengths of pipeline are well below the minimum run-up distance, it is then necessary to consider the probable magnitudes and durations of the pressures developed. Previous standard practice has consisted of attempts to define pressure histories in either the absence of confining walls or in the presence of walls of simple shape. Chapter 6 includes recent experimental studies of the interactions of detonations with complex shapes such as bends, junctions and contractions in area which invariably exist in chemical plant. These show clearly that wide variations in both the magnitude and duration of pressures occur locally. They are the result of the interactions of wave systems set up at expansive walls, (which result in quenching of reaction fronts), with those set up at compressive walls, which result in closer than normal coupling of the reaction zones and shock fronts. The process of reinitiation of quenched portions of the front apparently generates abnormally high pressures in a stochastic fashion. Consequently, although it is probably possible to stipulate a maximum pressure and a maximum duration, it is impossible to be precise about the location of such a pressure history. Whilst suites of computer programs are available for describing the response of structures to well-defined loading histories, for instance Bersafe [43, 44], their application to describing the effects of a detonation are apparently precluded. It appears that the common practice of assessing vulnerability of plant in terms of the relative magnitudes of the greatest pressure likely to be generated, and the static pressure which the plant will withstand, will continue. On the more positive side, the results described in Chapter 6 identify the general localities in which extremely high pressures are generated in complex components and should be of considerable assistance to accident investigations.

Chapter 7 is concerned with experimental studies of the strains and damage produced by confined detonations. The tests described were carried out in straight pipelines and measurements made at the side walls or at an end plate from which the detonation reflected normally. Probably, in misguided attempts to maximize pressures and resultant damage, the detonations were produced in stoichiometric mixtures of fuel and oxidant, and thus the effects of anomalously high pressures generated locally by the non-planar nature of the front in marginally-detonable mixtures were minimized. Again, analyses of the response of the structure have been based on highly idealized pressure histories. None the less, it appears that the damage caused to structures in which the velocity of the stress value is much higher than that of the detonation itself, does not exceed that predicted from considerations of its response to a static load. However, there are indications that damage is enhanced when the velocity of the stress wave in the wall is comparable with the detonation velocity. Finally, from the standpoint of investigations of damage in explosions in plant, we call attention to the complex modes of deformation which may be caused by the normal reflection of a detonation.

Whilst there may be only minor economic penalties in designing straight runs of pipeline to withstand the effects of a detonation, the same is not true of bends, junctions, reactor vessels, etc. Consequently, it will frequently be necessary to prevent the formation of a detonation, or at least to minimize its effects. Suitable procedures are described in Chapter 8. Methods of inhibiting or quenching flames propagating at normal burning velocities are described in detail in standard texts on combustion; consequently only general features are presently discussed, principally in terms of inhibitors such as halogenated hydrocarbons, which are also effective in quenching a detonation. Certain additives in powdered form, when present in high concentrations, have been found to suppress detonations [45]. However, the mechanisms involved are not clear and it would be dangerous to recommend their general application. The bulk of experimental studies of the quenching of detonation waves in pipelines suggest that the optimum technique consists of an expansion in area combined with some form of flame trap. Various forms of flame trap including packings and water sprays have been found to be effective [46–48]. Suppression in compact vessels is shown to be best achieved by triggered injection of halogenated hydrocarbons. A triggered barrier of a gas of high sonic velocity, such as helium, is suggested as a suitable method of mitigating the effects of a possible detonation in an unconfined cloud of vapour [49].

Information on both experimental and theoretical aspects of venting pressures produced by an accelerating flame, in the early stages of the growth of an explosion, is readily available in the literature. However, much of this is based on the idealization of symmetrical flow continuing throughout the process of relief of pressure. This idealization is seldom realized in practice, so that Chapter 8 concentrates on features, such as the growth of turbulence induced by unsymmetrical flow, which can reduce the efficiency of venting in suppressing explosions. A theoretical treatment of venting of detonations occurs in Chapter 6. Finally, it has been suggested that it may be possible to control detonations by a number of methods, for instance the use of an electrical field [50]. These are briefly mentioned in Chapter 8, indicating that a much better understanding of their mode of operation would be required before confident recommendations could be made on their application.

The final chapter summarizes the difficulties in predicting both the magnitude and location of peak pressures produced by a detonation in media close to the limits of detonability, particularly during their interaction with a change in shape of the confining walls. The obvious moral is that measures aimed at the prevention of a detonation are manifestly superior to attempts to design complex structures to contain the effects of a detonation.

Finally, advances in our understanding of the development of a detonation, of the interaction of a detonation with surrounding walls and of the effects of such interactions on containment walls have come from work in a wide range of disciplines. Consequently, there are severe difficulties in presenting a well-balanced account, especially in terms of the extent to which background material is discussed. A detailed treatment of each aspect is beyond the scope of the present text. We have recognized that there is a case for including the most pertinent features, for instance the interactions of shocks and blast waves in non-reactive media with changes in the shape of containment, in terms of appendixes. However, we have chosen to deal with this problem by an approach based on extensive referencing.

2

Unidimensional models

2.1 Introductory remarks

In contrast to other aspects of detonations, there is a large store of information available on unidimensional models. A large amount of information comes from studies of liquid and solid explosives and, although much is equally relevant to detonations in gaseous media, it is frequently too esoteric for inclusion in a text which emphasizes the significant role the structure of real fronts plays in their propagation and interactions with confinement. However, because of the importance of C–J theory in its wide ranging use for estimating the average properties of the front, it is essential that the main features of unidimensional theories be appreciated. This poses some problems in choosing which material of marginal practical interest to omit. The approach adopted here is biased towards brevity and relies on the ready availability of more borderline material in standard treatises on detonations [5–7].

The following section is concerned with the properties of the planar leading shock, associated with unidimensional models of detonation waves. It gives a brief outline of how the pressure, temperature and density ratios across the front are derived from considerations of conservation of mass, momentum and energy, showing how these ratios vary with the Mach number of the leading wave. Section 2.3 goes on to extend this analysis to the effects of the addition of energy behind the front. This leads naturally to the Chapman–Jouguet [20, 21] state, described in Section 2.4. Section 2.5 contains the results of predictions of velocities of detonation waves and how they vary with parameters, such as composition of the mixture, obtained from widely-available computer programs based on C–J theory [29–31]. These are compared with typical experimental results, illustrating how well the theory performs in predicting average velocities. Nevertheless, a central assumption of C–J theory (that considerations of chemical equilibria, rather than chemical kinetics, govern the flow field behind the precursor shock) is untenable, so the more realistic model of Zel'dovich [22], von Neumann [23] and Doring [24] is described in Section 2.6. This model involves a delay between the passage of the precursor shock and the onset of exothermic chemical reactions. The logarithm of the delay exhibits an inverse exponential dependence on the temperature of the shock flow. The following section describes the performance of the ZND model in predicting pressures, densities and the properties of reaction zones in near-to-stoichiometric mixtures of fuel and oxidant. In order to define the shape of the tails of pressure profiles produced by both confined and unconfined detonations, and how they vary with distance from the origin of the front, the theory of the Taylor expansion front [51] is given in Section 2.8. The final section attempts to summarize the likely magnitude of errors in the prediction of properties, other than the average velocity, of detonations propagating along straight and smooth-walled ducts.

2.2 Properties of unidimensional shock waves

Common to all unidimensional models of detonation waves is a description based on a precursor shock followed closely by a coupled reaction zone. Furthermore, the velocity of the leading shock for both confined and unconfined detonations is generally assumed to be constant in a mixture of given chemical composition and of uniform initial temperature and pressure. Indeed, as we shall see, there is much experimental evidence on confined detonations supporting this contention. Consequently, before considering the effects of the addition of chemical energy to the flow behind the front, it is logical to begin with a description of the laws governing the properties of a steady shock front in a non-reactive medium. By initially neglecting the details of the chemical kinetics connected with the addition of energy, it is possible to highlight the essential gasdynamic phenomena.

Consider a planar shock front propagating at a steady velocity W_s into quiescent inert gas, as depicted in Fig. 2.1(a). Assume that the properties of the gas jump discontinuously at the front, but have steady values in the regions

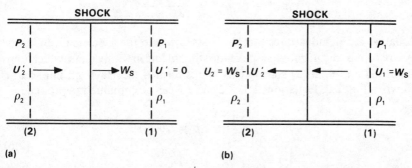

Figure 2.1 Non-reactive planar shock (a) in laboratory-fixed and (b) shock-fixed co-ordinates.

ahead and behind the wave, defined by the two control surfaces (1) and (2) parallel to the front. Pressure, density and velocity of the gas are denoted by p, ρ and u respectively. It is possible to simplify the analysis by transforming to a coordinate system with an origin fixed at the shock front to replace a laboratory frame of reference. The resulting flows are shown in Fig. 2.1(b). Here the gas flows into the stationary shock front with a velocity W_s and emerges from the front with a velocity $u_2 = W_s - u_2'$, where u_2' is the velocity of the gas relative to a stationary observer. Although the processes which occur in the vicinity of the shock front are irreversible, the three mechanical conservation conditions apply rigorously to the flows through the control surfaces. In integral form they may be expressed as

conservation of mass $\qquad \rho_1 W_s = \rho_2 u_2$ $\qquad\qquad$ (2.1)

conservation of momentum $\quad p_1 + \rho_1 W_s^2 = p_2 + \rho_2 u_2^2$ $\qquad$ (2.2)

and

conservation of energy $\qquad h_1 + \dfrac{1}{2} W_s^2 = h_2 + \dfrac{1}{2} u_2^2$ $\qquad$ (2.3)

where $h = e + pv$ is the specific enthalpy, e is the internal energy and $v = 1/\rho$ is the specific volume. Furthermore, for the strengths of shocks typical of detonation, the ideal equation of state for a gas can generally be assumed to hold:

$$p = \rho RT \qquad\qquad (2.4)$$

where R is the gas constant. Equations 2.1–2.4 have five unknown quantities, W_s, u_2, ρ_2, p_2 and T_2, so that all the properties of the post-shock flow in region 2 can be expressed in terms of the velocity of the front and the initial conditions of the gas.

Equations 2.1 and 2.2 give an expression for the mass flow through the shock, ρ, thus

$$(W_s \rho_1)^2 = (u_2 \rho_2)^2 = \frac{(p_2 - p_1)}{(v_1 - v_2)} \qquad\qquad (2.5)$$

Equation 2.5 demonstrates that the mass flow into the shock is given by the square root of the negative slope of the straight line in the pv plane which joins initial (1) and final (2) states. This line is termed the Rayleigh line, and is shown in Fig. 2.2. Equations 2.1, 2.2 and 2.3 can be combined to produce

$$h_2 - h_1 = \frac{1}{2}(p_2 - p_1)(v_1 + v_2)$$

or $\qquad\qquad\qquad\qquad\qquad\qquad\qquad\qquad\qquad\qquad\qquad\qquad$ (2.6)

$$e_2 - e_1 = \frac{1}{2}(p_2 + p_1)(v_1 - v_2)$$

Equation 2.6 is denoted the Rankine–Hugoniot, R–H, relationship, occasionally and regrettably shortened to the Hugoniot relationship. It characterizes the initial and final states resulting from a given change in energy or enthalpy across the shock front. In other words, it is the counterpart of the relationship for isentropic and adiabatic processes $de = -p \, dv$, or $pv^\gamma = $ constant. The curves are shown in the typical $p - v$ diagram, Fig. 2.2.

Assuming that there is no change in specific heat ratio and molecular weight of the gas, Equations 2.1 to 2.4 can be combined to yield pressure, density and

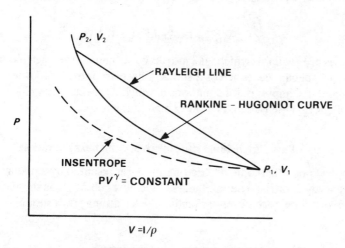

Figure 2.2   Rankine-Hugoniot p–v relationship (Rayleigh line).

temperature ratios across the front in terms of its Mach number, $M_s = W_s/a_1$, where a_1 is the speed of sound in the medium ahead of the shock (Equations 2.7, 2.8 and 2.9).

$$p_2/p_1 = p_{21} = \frac{2\gamma M_s^2 - (\gamma - 1)}{(\gamma + 1)} \tag{2.7}$$

$$\rho_2/\rho_1 = \rho_{21} = \frac{(\gamma + 1)M_s^2}{(\gamma - 1)M_s^2 + 2} \tag{2.8}$$

$$T_2/T_1 = T_{21} = \frac{\left[\gamma M_s^2 - \dfrac{(\gamma - 1)}{2}\right]\left[\dfrac{(\gamma - 1)}{2}M_s^2 + 1\right]}{\dfrac{\gamma + 1}{2}M_s^2} \tag{2.9}$$

As will become apparent shortly, detonation waves in gaseous mixtures at initial pressures of about a bar and initial temperatures of about 300 K are characterized by leading fronts with Mach numbers $4 \leq M_D \leq 8$. Hence, the following approximations hold to the degree of accuracy required of most design studies

$$p_{21} \simeq \frac{2\gamma M_D^2}{\gamma+1}, \, \rho_{21} \simeq \frac{\gamma+1}{\gamma-1} \text{and } T_{21} \simeq \frac{\gamma(\gamma-1)}{(\gamma+1)^2} M_D^2 \qquad (2.10)$$

For a gas mixture with a constant value of $\gamma = 1.4$, approximated to by fuel-lean mixtures with air, the following approximations are satisfactory for $M_D \geq 4$:

$$p_{21} \simeq 1.2 M_D^2, \, \rho_{21} \simeq 6 \text{ and } T_{21} \simeq 0.2 M_D^2 \qquad (2.11)$$

Analyses are available which take into account changes in molecular weight and ratio of specific heats across a shock. These are introduced later in this Chapter and in Chapter 6, for situations in which it is necessary to include the effects of energy released in the flow behind the shock.

2.3 Properties of unidimensional shock waves with energy addition

The simplest possible model of a detonation is represented by a planar shock with an energy addition q per unit mass of the flow behind it (as shown in Fig. 2.3 in a coordinate system, rendering the shock stationary). It should perhaps

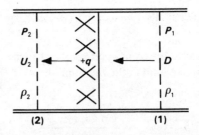

Figure 2.3 Planar shock with exothermic reaction and steady flow in shock-fixed coordinates.

be emphasized that this does not purport to be a physically-meaningful description of a detonation, but rather a model which emphasizes the fluid dynamic aspects of the process. Then, of the conservation equations applying to a non-reactive front, only that for energy, Equation 2.3, is modified and becomes

$$h_2 - h_1 - q = \frac{1}{2}(p_2 - p_1)(v_1 + v_2) \qquad (2.12)$$

For an ideal gas of constant γ Equation 2.12 can be rewritten as

$$\frac{\gamma}{(\gamma-1)}(p_2 v_2 - p_1 v_1) - q = \frac{1}{2}(p_2 - p_1)(v_1 + v_2) \qquad (2.13)$$

When the final states of the R–H equation appropriately modified for addition of energy (2.12) are plotted on a p–v plane, with q as the variable parameter, a family of rectangular hyperbolae result. Two such curves corresponding with a non-reactive shock, $q = 0$ and a finite value of q, are

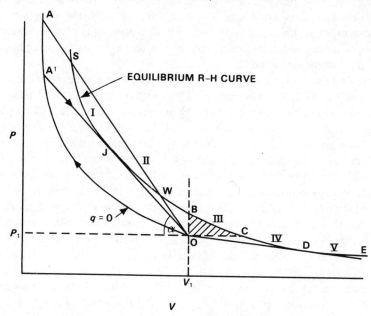

Figure 2.4 Influence of energy addition, q, on Rankine–Hugoniot curves.

shown in Fig. 2.4. In order to describe the various possible solutions to Equation 2.12, it is useful to consider the final or equilibrium R–H consisting of five regions. These are obtained by drawing the two tangents from point O (representing the initial conditions p and v) to the curve, and by constructing two lines of $p = $ constant and $v = $ constant through O. The resulting portions SJ, JB, BC, CD and DE are labelled by the Roman numerals I to V on Fig. 2.4.

For simplicity, first consider region III. Here $p_2 > p_1$ and $v_2 > v_1$, so that (from Equation 2.5, giving the shock velocity in terms of p and v):

$$W_s = \left[\frac{(p_2 - p_1)}{(v_1 - v_2)}\right]^{1/2} = \tan\alpha \qquad (2.14)$$

W_s is imaginary and consequently region III does not correspond to a real situation of flow. Regions I and II correspond to the detonation branch of the R–H curve. On AJBC, $p_2 > p_1$ and $v_2 < v_1$, so that the final states correspond to a compressive shock in both regions I and II. The properties of this branch are most readily described by constructing a secant through O, which intersects the final R–H curve at S and W. For a given velocity of wave W_s, defined by the slope, $\tan \alpha$, of the secant, there are in general two solutions for the end states S and W. The solution corresponding to S is the higher pressure and consequently is referred to as a strong detonation, whereas that corresponding to W is denoted a weak detonation. The possibility that two detonation velocities are realizable is at variance with the experimental observation that the detonation velocity is unique for a given gaseous medium. Consequently, it is necessary to examine more deeply the physical significance of regions I and II.

In region I the sum of sound speed and gas velocity is greater than the wave velocity $(a + u > D)$; thus the velocity of flow with respect to the leading shock is subsonic. Then, any rarefaction arising in the flow behind the leading wave will eventually overtake and weaken it. The resultant decrease in velocity of the shock shifts the end state towards J. In contrast, in region II the sum of sound speed and flow velocity is less than the velocity of the front $(a + u < D)$, so that the velocity of the flow is supersonic with respect to the front. Thus, the chemical energy assumed to have been released in a steady zone is, in fact, released in a non-steady region, and, as a result, is not available to support the shock front. In consequence the velocity of the front again falls to approach point J, therefore J represents the only stable end state for which the release of chemical energy in the shocked flow allows the sustenance of the leading shock. The gradient of the tangent drawn from the initial state, O to J represents the minimum velocity of front compatible with the conservation laws. This is the form in which Chapman [20] first stated his hypothesis, which, following Jouguet's [21] investigation of the uniqueness of such a solution, became embodied in the celebrated Chapman–Jouguet hypothesis (namely $a + u_2 = D$). Alternatively, a self-sustaining detonation requires the existence of a plane, parallel to and behind the front, at which equilibrium exists and where the flow, relative to the front, is sonic. This boundary is denoted the Chapman–Jouguet plane.

In regions IV and V of the equilibrium R–H curve, the final states are below the initial values $p_2 < p_1$ and $v_2 < v_1$. They represent a deflagration wave in which a rarefaction fan travels behind a combustion front. It can be demonstrated that the condition for a line to be drawn from O to be a tangent to the lower branch of the R–H curve at D is similar to that for the tangent to the upper branch OJ, i.e. the velocity of the flow of burnt gas relative to the front must be sonic. Both types of steady flow are termed Chapman–Jouguet flows, and the tangent points J and D termed upper and lower Chapman–Jouguet points. However, our principal concern here is the detonation branch of the R–H curve which is now considered in greater detail.

2.4 Properties of the Chapman–Jouguet state

Having established that, for a stable complex (consisting of a shock wave and reaction zone in steady unidimensional flow), the C–J condition holds for one end state p_2, v_2 only of those defined by the R–H equation, it is possible to examine the properties of the C–J condition in more detail. By eliminating the pressure ratio across the shock, p_{21} (from Equations 2.13 and 2.5)

$$v_{21} = p_{12} = \frac{1 + \gamma M^2 \pm \left[(M^2 - 1)^2 - \frac{2(\gamma + 1)(\gamma - 1)M^2 q}{a_1^2} \right]^{1/2}}{(\gamma + 1)M^2} \qquad (2.15)$$

Equation 2.15, as expected, defines two end states, and the C–J condition is obtained by setting the radical equal to zero, when

$$\frac{\gamma - 1}{a_1^2} q_{max} = \frac{(M^2 - 1)^2}{2(\gamma + 1)M^2} \qquad (2.16)$$

This defines the maximum amount of energy that can be added to the flow associated with a precursor shock of specified Mach number. As such, it represents the addition of energy required for unidimensional, steady and choked flow. Hence, q_{max} can be equated with q_{CJ}, so that

$$q_{CJ} = \frac{a_1^2}{(\gamma - 1)} \frac{(M_{CJ}^2 - 1)^2}{2(\gamma + 1)M_{CJ}^2} \qquad (2.17)$$

This is shown graphically in Fig. 2.5, as a plot of the flow velocity relative to the shock front, u, versus the energy addition q. Two values of u exist for each value of q; one representing supersonic and the other subsonic flow. The maximum value of q corresponds with a flow Mach number of unity, which is the C–J condition.

We can now consider how to calculate the C–J properties of a given detonable medium. The calculation involves the solution of: (a) the three conservation equations, (b) the equation describing the C–J condition, (c) the equation of state of the products of reaction, and (d) those describing thermal equilibrium. It can be shown that, at the C–J point, the gradient of the R–H curve is also that of the isentrope

$$\left(\frac{dp_2}{dv_2} \right)_{R\text{-}H} = \left(\frac{dp_2}{dv_2} \right)_S \qquad (2.18)$$

so that

$$\frac{\gamma_2 p_2}{v_2} = \frac{p_2 - p_1}{v_1 - v_2} \qquad (2.19)$$

where S denotes entropy.

Thus, a combination of Equations 2.13 and 2.19 allows the properties of the front to be determined, providing that the effective energy release, q, at the C–J plane is known. Using readily available thermochemical data to obtain equilibrium concentrations of products (and hence q and γ_2), the conditions obtaining at the C–J plane may be evaluated with great precision [29–31]. The appropriate thermochemical data have been incorporated in a number of computer programs for the solution of Equations 2.13 and 2.19 and these are now almost universally used to calculate the properties of the front. Little purpose would be served by including a detailed description of their operation

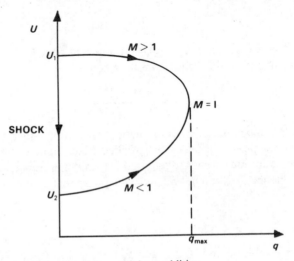

Figure 2.5   Uni-dimensional flow with heat addition.

here. However, it may be useful to include some typical examples of their performance. Figure 2.6 illustrates how the nature of the fuel molecule influences the variation in predicted C–J velocity with the composition of the mixture of fuel and oxygen. The computations have been carried out between the experimentally-determined limits for spherical detonations in these mixtures. Note the similarities in slope of the curves for fuel-lean mixtures of molecules of similar ratios of hydrogen to carbon atoms. Figure 2.7 is a similar plot, showing the effects of changing the oxidant from oxygen to air in mixtures of *n*-butane with the oxidant. In this case the computations have been extended between the composition limits for confined detonations. We shall expand on this in Chapter 4; however, at this stage it is worth noting that there is no apparent relationship between the C–J velocities at the upper and lower limits of detonability. Finally, Fig. 2.8 illustrates the predicted effect of increasing concentration of a diluent (in this case nitrogen) on reducing the C–J velocity in two self-decomposing fuels, acetylene and ozone. The equilibrium composition of the products of the diluted ozone detonation includes significant amounts of nitrogen oxides, possibly accounting for the differences in rates of attenuation of the C–J velocities at high degrees of dilution.

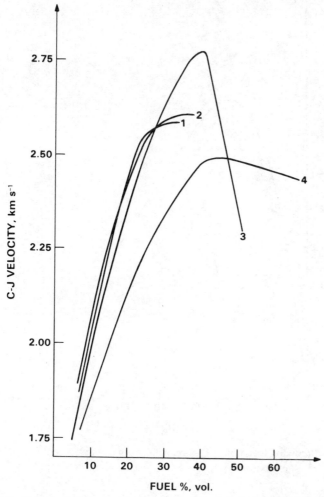

Figure 2.6 Predicted C–J velocities in mixtures of various fuels with oxygen [31]. (1) propane; (2) propene; (3) propadiene and methylacetylene and (4) ethylene oxide.

In many instances an approximate estimate of the flow conditions associated with a C–J wave suffices. Since typically $M_{CJ} \geq 4$ the following approximations are both useful and reasonably accurate:

$$p_2 \approx \frac{2q(\gamma_2 - 1)}{v_1} \qquad \frac{v_2}{v_1} = \frac{\rho_1}{\rho_2} = \frac{\gamma_1}{\gamma_1 + 1}$$

$$T_2 \approx \frac{2q\gamma_2}{(\gamma_2 + 1)a_2} \qquad u_2 = \left[\frac{2q(\gamma_2 - 1)}{(\gamma_2 + 1)}\right]^{1/2}$$

$$D \approx [2q(\gamma_2{}^2 - 1)]^{1/2} \tag{2.20}$$

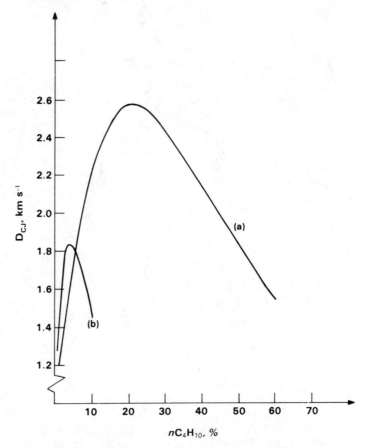

Figure 2.7 Predicted variation in C–J velocities with composition of (a) n-C_4H_{10}–O_2 and (b) n-C_4H_{10}–air mixtures [31].

In addition,

$$D = \frac{\gamma_2 + 1}{\gamma_2} a_2 \text{ and } u_2 = \frac{a_2}{\gamma_2}$$

From these it is easy to show that if p_v and T_v are the pressure and temperature reached in an explosion at constant volume, then

$$T_2/T_v \simeq 2\gamma_2/(\gamma_2 + 1) \text{ and } p_2/p_v \sim 2.$$

2.5 Comparison of C–J predictions and experiment

There have been frequent attempts to verify the C–J hypothesis experimentally, the majority of which have involved a comparison of the wave velocity of confined detonations with the theoretical value. Although velocity

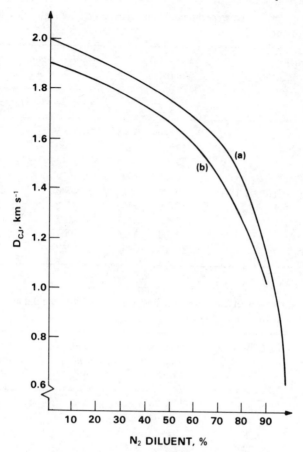

Figure 2.8   The effect of nitrogen as a diluent in reducing predicted C–J velocities in self-decomposing media [31]. (a) $C_2H_2 + N_2$ and (b) $O_3 + N_2$.

is the parameter most easily measured with high precision, it has a number of drawbacks as a yardstick. For instance, since it is theoretically proportional to the slope of the tangent to the equilibrium R–H curve from the initial state, it is somewhat insensitive to the properties assumed for the final states. Again, in early tests of the theory, inaccurate thermochemical data were used in computing velocities. Finally, in order to account for losses to the wall, the experimental studies need to be conducted in tubes of different diameters and extrapolated to a velocity in a tube of infinite diameter, with which to compare the theoretical value.

An early study was of stoichiometric mixtures of oxygen and acetylene diluted with various inert gases [52]. The agreement between measured and theoretical velocities of the front, shown in Table 2.1, is better than 10% over

Table 2.1 Comparison of experimental and calculated C–J velocities in diluted oxyhydrogen mixtures [8].

Explosive mixture	p_2 (atm.)	T_2 (K)	Detonation velocity (ms^{-1})	
			Calculated	Experimental
$(2H_2 + O_2)$	18.05	3583	2086	2819
$(2H_2 + O_2) + 1.5He$	17.60	3412	3200	3010
$(2H_2 + O_2) + 3He$	17.11	3265	3432	3130
$(2H_2 + O_2) + 5He$	16.32	3097	3613	3160
$(2H_2 + O_2) + (2.82He + 1.18Ar)$	16.68	3175	2620	2390
$(2H_2 + O_2) + (1.5He + 1.5Ar)$	17.11	3265	2356	2330
$(2H_2 + O_2) + 1.5Ar$	17.60	3412	2117	1950
$(2H_2 + O_2) + 3Ar$	17.11	3265	1907	1800
$(2H_2 + O_2) + 5Ar$	16.32	3097	1762	1700

Table 2.2 Comparison of experimental and C–J velocities calculated from more accurate thermochemical data [54].

Mixture	Observed velocity (ms^{-1})	Theoretical velocity (ms^{-1})	Standard deviation (%)	Deviation from theory (%)
$4H_2 + O_2$	3344	3425	0.7	−2.3
$3H_2 + O_2$	3156	3197	0.2	−1.3
$2H_2 + O_2$	2825	2853	0.5	−1.0
$H_2 + O_2$	2320	2333	0.5	−0.6
$H_2 + 2O_2$	1909	1941	0.3	−1.6
$H_2 + 3O_2$	1691	1759	0.3	−3.8

a wide range of dilutions. A reassessment of the theoretical values using more accurate thermochemical data resulted in improved agreement, to better than ±2%.

Further examples of velocity measurements in a 100 mm diameter tube, compared with predictions which are again based on improved chemical data [53, 54], are shown in Table 2.2. The measured velocities, as might be expected taking into account losses to the wall, are consistently lower than the theoretical values, with a maximum deviation of 3.8%.

Although agreement between theory and experiment for stoichiometric mixtures appears impressively good, it is generally accepted that the theory considerably overestimates velocities in mixtures nearer to the limits of detonability. Typically, the predicted velocity can be up to 30% greater than

Table 2.3 Theoretical and measured pressures in oxyhydrogen mixtures [54].

Mixture	Observed peak pressure (atm.)	Non-equilibrium theory peak pressure (atm.)	Observed average pressure 20–80 μs (atm.)	Theoretical C–J pressure (atm.)
$4H_2 + O_2$	27.3	32.69	18.0	17.78
$3H_2 + O_2$	28.1	33.89	18.4	18.44
$2H_2 + O_2$	27.1	34.16	18.6	18.59
$H_2 + O_2$	26.1	32.43	18.3	17.63
$H_2 + 2O_2$	25.0	29.10	16.7	15.79
$H_2 + 3O_2$	24.9	26.06	15.1	14.14

the measured value [55]. Bearing this and previous provisos about the use of velocity as a yardstick in mind, it would be reassuring to have comparisons with other parameters. Table 2.3 shows a comparison of predicted and measured pressures [54]. Pressure measurements are bedevilled by difficulties in ensuring that the response time of the transducer is adequate, so that some form of time-averaging is generally necessary. The first and second columns of the table show a comparison of measured and theoretical peak pressures. These are considerably higher than the C–J levels shown in the final column, and have to be accounted for in terms of a non-equilibrium von Neumann spike (second column). Whilst the averaged pressures measured over the period 20–80 μs are in reasonably close accord with the C–J predictions, the existence of the non-equilibrium peak calls attention to the dangers of basing the design of plant on C–J theory.

2.6 The Zel'dovich, von Neumann, Doring model

It is unquestionable that the simple model based on the ideas of Chapman and Jouguet was successful in predicting the average velocities of detonations. Even with the approximate thermochemical data available in the 1930s, early predictions of velocities were of acceptable accuracy. With the advent of more refined thermodynamic data, the discrepancies between theory and experiment were reduced to less than 2%. It is frequently suggested that the noted successes of the simple hydrodynamic model were instrumental in delaying a critical examination of the structure of the front. Thus, although it was known that complex three-dimensional effects such as spin were manifested by detonations in marginally-detonable media confined in tubes, the simple unidimensional theory was assumed to hold for waves in more detonable media. It was not until Zel'dovich [22], von Neumann [23] and Doring [24] independently proposed their models, that the realistic concept of finite rates of chemical reaction was introduced into a description of detonation fronts, and it became possible to account quantitatively for features such as velocity deficits in terms of losses from the flow regime behind the precursor front.

In its simplest guise, the ZND model assumes the flow is unidimensional and not subject to viscous losses. Again, the leading shock is treated as a discontinuity but, in contrast to the C–J model, no reaction occurs in the flow immediately behind the shock. The reaction follows an incubation period, during which a pool of chemically-active species is formed at a finite rate at the high temperature and pressure of the shocked medium. The reaction is represented by a single forward-rate process, gradually progressing to completion some distance behind the precursor shock. The extent of reaction is measured in terms of a reaction coordinate, ξ, which has the value 0 immediately behind the front and unity at the plane at which reaction is complete.

Applying the conservation equations 2.1, 2.2 and 2.12 between the control plane 1 and a plane characterized by the fraction ξ, where the energy released is $q\xi$, gives a corresponding R–H curve. Thus, for each plane there is an R–H curve, and the complete reaction zone is described by a family of R–H curves.

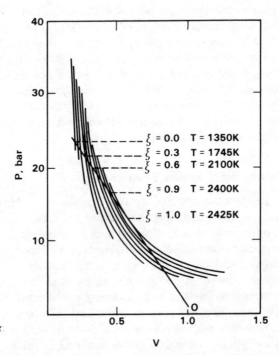

Figure 2.9 Family of R–H curves corresponding to successive tenths of fraction reacted, ξ, in 20% H_2–air mixtures, with O representing initial conditions (after Gordon [56]).

An example of such a family for the reaction in a mixture of 20% hydrogen in air is shown in Fig. 2.9 [56]. The curves show how the pressure varies with the degree of energy released within the reaction zone in which ξ increases from zero to unity. In order to obtain the temporal variation in pressure a detailed knowledge of the rates of the various reactions is required.

Before discussing the nature of the reaction zone incorporated in the ZND model, it is worth emphasizing that this more realistic representation is still combined with an essentially steady and unidimensional model of the flow. Since the end state of the reaction is that of the C–J model, the C–J hypothesis is still applicable and the C–J velocity is independent of the rate law chosen to describe the rate of reaction.

The simplest concept of the reaction zone associated with a unidimensional front comes from an analogy with the processes occurring in normal flames at, or below, atmospheric pressure. It involves the predication of an induction zone in the flow immediately behind the leading shock. Here, chemically active species are produced by fast bimolecular steps in which one radical attacking a molecular species results in the formation of two radicals (chain-branching). Overall, the processes in this region are thermoneutral. In the flow some distance behind the induction zone is the recombination zone, in which the chemical energy is liberated in a series of three-body reaction steps, where neutral species serve to carry off the heat of association of the product molecules. These three-body steps eventually result in a mixture at chemical equilibrium at the C–J plane. The chemical kinetics are best described in terms of the hydrogen–oxygen system, which has been exhaustively investigated and for which reliable data on the rates of individual steps exist. The important steps are as follows:

Initiation	H_2 or $O_2 + M \rightarrow 2H^{\bullet}$ or $2O^{\bullet} + M$	(2.21)
Chain branching	$H^{\bullet} + O_2 \rightarrow OH^{\bullet} + O^{\bullet}$	(2.22)
	$O^{\bullet} + H_2 \rightarrow OH^{\bullet} + H^{\bullet}$	(2.23)
Recombination	$H^{\bullet} + H^{\bullet} + M \rightarrow H_2 + M$	(2.24)
	$O^{\bullet} + O^{\bullet} + M \rightarrow O_2 + M$	(2.25)
	$H^{\bullet} + OH^{\bullet} + M \rightarrow H_2O + M$	(2.26)

In order to characterize the induction zone by a time τ, the simplest assumptions possible is that the overall rate is controlled by a highly endothermic and slow step (Equation 2.21). More commonly, and more accurately, τ is related to the temperature T and density ρ of the shocked gas by an Arrhenius expression of the form

$$\ln[O_2]\tau = \frac{A}{\rho^n} \exp(E_a/RT)$$

(2.27)

where $[O_2]$ is the concentration of oxygen, R the gas constant and E_a a temperature coefficient well below that of the reaction step in Equation 2.21. At the close of the induction period, the rapid bimolecular reactions (Equations 2.22 and 2.23) are in equilibrium, but the slower 3-body processes (Equations 2.24 to 2.26) are not. However, the resultant mixture may be regarded as being in a state of partial equilibrium, so that a single recombination parameter suffices to describe the progress of the reaction to a state of full equilibrium.

In order to avoid possible confusion, it is worth noting that some authors, when referring to the reaction zone or the combustion wave, imply the recombination zone only, since it is the region in which chemical energy is released. This energy can be communicated to the leading shock by pressure waves, because the gas flow is subsonic relative to the front.

2.7 Comparison of the ZND model and experiment

From 1950 to 1970 considerable effort was expended in attempts to test the range of validity of the ZND model. As with similar tests of the C–J model, attention was focussed on highly accurate measurements of the wave velocity. Summarizing the results of such work, the observed velocities of fronts in near-to-stoichiometric mixtures confined in straight tubes with smooth walls were found to deviate from predicted values by amounts greater than the uncertainties in the best available experimental data. Fay [25] was able to show that the magnitude of the deficit in velocity, ΔW_d, was consistent with the presence of a wall boundary layer behind the front. His analysis formed the basis for the formula commonly used to deduce the velocity of a front in a tube of infinite diameter

$$\frac{\Delta W_d}{W_d} = \frac{2.1\delta}{d} \tag{2.28}$$

where δ is a function of the thickness of the boundary layer and d the diameter of the tube. Further studies showed that whilst corrected values of velocity were most frequently still slightly below the C–J value, they were occasionally greater [57]. This anomaly must call into question whether the effects of a boundary layer are the sole cause of the departure from theory. It is worth emphasizing that the discrepancies between theory and experiment are less than 1%, so their implications to the design of plant are minimal.

A limited amount of work has been done in comparing experimental pressure histories with those predicted by the ZND model. However, the stringent demands made on the performance of pressure gauges (in terms of testing the C–J model) will be recalled. Thus, for mixtures of fuel and oxygen of near-stoichiometric composition and at atmospheric pressure, the duration of the reaction zones is only a few microseconds. Although it is possible to broaden the reaction zone by reducing the initial pressure or by the addition of an inert diluent, such measures result in the generation of oscillations of large amplitude, making it difficult to deduce what is the average pressure profile. In general, it has been necessary to compromise between acceptable spatial resolution and degree of oscillatory perturbations. An example of the profile of a 'side-on' or static pressure in a stoichiometric oxyhydrogen mixture at an initial pressure of 100 torr [54] is shown in Fig. 2.10 with that predicted by the ZND model. Possibly on account of damping of the response of the gauge, there are no indications of pressure oscillations typical of transverse fronts on the experimental record. Figure 3.10 shows a pressure history more typical of those likely to be obtained in near-limit mixtures, showing the complexities in interpreting the further peaks produced by

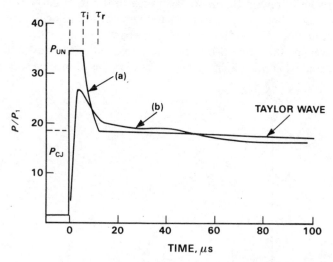

Figure 2.10 Idealized ZND pressure profile (a) and experimental profile (b) in $2H_2 + O_2$ mixture at $p_0 = 100$ torr. τ_i induction zone; τ_r recombination zone.

transverse waves. The predicted history shows the frontal shock followed by a region of constant pressure, in which the thermoneutral chain-branching reactions occur (von Neumann spike). After this peak the recombination reactions result in a rapid decrease in pressure which continues to the C–J plane, at which they cease. Finally, there is the Taylor expansion wave, the head of which is at the C–J plane. The properties of this are described in Section 2.8.

   In comparing the experimental and model histories of pressure, there are three points to note. First, even after due allowance for limitations in the response of the gauge, the amplitude of the observed peak is less than that of the theoretical prediction. That this is generally true can be seen from the values for the two peaks given in Table 2.3. Second, after the experimental initial peak there is a plateau, and third, the observed onset of the Taylor expansion wave is apparently delayed. This could well be accounted for, should the actual flow be supersonic rather than subsonic, relative to the front, as required by the model.

Precise measurements of the density versus time characteristics of detonations, as with pressure are fraught with considerable experimental difficulties. However, they do offer the potential advantage of high spatial resolution. Two studies have used the absorption of X-rays [58] and inter-ferometry [59] to monitor the density of the mixture behind detonation fronts to an estimated accuracy of ±1%. Both studies suggested that, even after making due allowance for the effects of boundary layers, the measured density was as much as 15% below the predicted value. This indicates that detonations lie in region II, the weak branch of the R–H curve (Fig. 2.4). Confirmation of this comes from measurements of the velocity of the flow behind detonations. These have employed spark sources with a schlieren system to record the angle β between the direction of the flow and Mach waves, created by accidental irregularities in the walls of the test section [60,

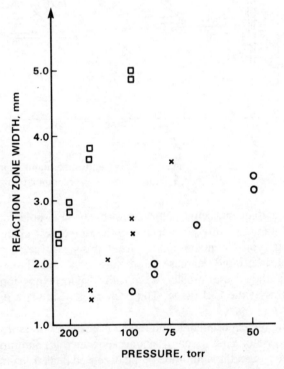

Figure 2.11 Variation in thickness of reaction zone with initial composition and pressure, after Wagner [62]. %–Hexane, □ 6%; ○ 9.5%; × 16%.

61]. The local Mach number of the flow, M', is then defined by $M' = 1/\sin\beta$. For mixtures of various compositions of hydrogen and oxygen typical values were found to lie in the range $1.2 \le M' \le 1.4$.

Finally, some discrepancies in the results of detailed studies of the widths of the reaction zones in mixtures of oxygen and hydrogen and of oxygen [62] and various hydrocarbons [62, 63], appeared to have been resolved; showing that the reaction zones are considerably thicker than unidimensional theories suggest, possibly by a factor of up to ten [63]. Differences of this magnitude must cast considerable doubt on the validity of pressure profiles deduced from unidimensional theories. Figure 2.11 shows how the observed thickness of the combined induction and recombination regions in mixtures of *n*-hexane with oxygen vary with initial pressure and fuel content of the mixtures. Although the experimental values of thickness of reaction zone depend on initial pressure and composition of the mixture, the observed variations are more complex than are suggested by unidimensional theory (equation 2.27).

In summary, unidimensional models of detonations perform satisfactorily in predicting average detonation velocities in readily detonable mixtures confined in smooth-walled tubes. As we shall see in the following Chapter on the structure of real detonations, they can only give general guidance on the average velocities to be expected in less ideal systems, or on the probable variation across a front. More importantly, pressures and densities of the shocked flow derived from such velocities may well be as much as 15% too low, even in idealized systems.

2.8 The Taylor expansion wave

Although the centred expansion fan, following the reaction zone, is not strictly a part of either the C–J or ZND models, it is appropriate at this stage to include a description of some of its properties. In particular, we shall consider how the tail of the pressure profile, exerted by detonations propagating through straight and either closed or open-ended tube, varies with distance from the point of initiation. Since the leading edge of the Taylor expansion is located at the C–J plane, a brief recapitulation of the factors influencing its position may be helpful. It will be recalled that the C–J plane is that at which the flow becomes sonic with respect to the shock; hence, its position is defined differently by the two unidimensional theories. For C–J theory, it is given by the mechanism assumed to govern the expansion of the products; for ZND theory the width of the reaction zone must first be estimated. On the assumption that the subsequent expansion from the pressure and temperature calculated from standard unidimensional theory is isentropic, it is then possible to use the analysis presently outlined.

The product gases beyond the C–J plane continue to accelerate as they expand isentropically, causing their temperature and pressure to continue to fall. Taylor [51] was the first to examine in detail the distribution of velocities in this non-steady regime. By assuming that the exothermic recombination reactions are completed upstream, that the subsequent flow is isentropic and that dissipative effects are absent, the change in velocity of the gas behind planar fronts is related to its change in density by

$$u - u_2 = \int_{\rho}^{\rho_2} a \frac{d\rho}{\rho} \tag{2.29}$$

and since the speed of sound, a, is given by

$$a = a_2 \left(\frac{\rho}{\rho_2} \right)^{(\gamma - 1)/2} \tag{2.30}$$

then

$$u = u_2 - \frac{2a_2}{\gamma - 1} \left[1 - \left(\frac{\rho}{\rho_2} \right)^{(\gamma - 1)/2} \right]$$

or

$$\tag{2.31}$$

$$u = u_2 - \frac{2a_2}{\gamma - 1} \left[1 - \left(\frac{p}{p_2} \right)^{(\gamma - 1)/2\gamma} \right]$$

Hence

$$u + a = u_2 + a_2 - \left(\frac{\gamma + 1}{2} \right)(u_2 - u) \tag{2.32}$$

Consider now a detonation confined in a straight tube, where there are two possible boundary conditions at the end the front originates, $x = 0$. With the tube open at this end $u + a = 0$, so that Equation 2.32 yields

$$u_0 = u_2 - \left(\frac{2}{\gamma + 1} \right)(u_2 + a_2) \tag{2.33}$$

With a closed end $u = 0$, and Equation 2.32 becomes

$$a = u_2 + a_2 - \left(\frac{\gamma + 1}{2} \right)u_2 = \left(\frac{1 - \gamma}{2} \right)u_2 + a_2 \tag{2.34}$$

Thus, the decay in gas velocity with distance behind the front, $x = (u + a)t$ can be obtained. Taking values typical of a C–J wave $u \approx \frac{1}{3}D_{CJ}$, $a = \frac{2}{3}D_{CJ}$ and $\gamma \approx 1.3$, the result for an open-ended tube is given in Fig. 2.12. Point C in Fig. 2.12 represents the exit velocity in an open-ended tube with an external pressure of zero, the negative value indicating that the direction of flow is opposite to that of the front. If, as usual, there is a finite counter-pressure at the open end, then a steady velocity of flow is attained somewhere between the point 0 and $x = 0$. The point A, from which gas is at rest, to $x = 0$ in a tube with closed end can be found by manipulation of Equation 2.34. Thus

$$\frac{a}{D_{CJ}} = \frac{u_2 + a_2}{D_{CJ}} - \left(\frac{\gamma + 1}{2}\right)\frac{u_2}{D_{CJ}} = 1 - \frac{a_2(\gamma + 1)}{2D_{CJ}} \tag{2.35}$$

Again using values typical of a C–J front, the ratio $x/X = 0.616$, where X is the distance of the detonation front from $x = 0$.

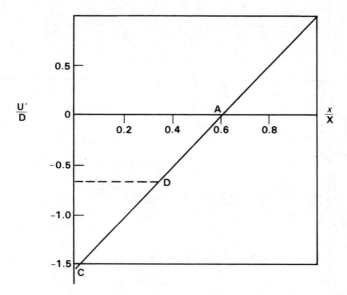

Figure 2.12 Distribution of velocities behind planar detonation fronts $p\rho^{-1.3} = $ constant after Taylor [51].

It may be useful to note the following relationships, derived from Equation 2.30, for the decay in pressure and temperature of the flow in a Taylor expansion behind a detonation in a straight tube

$$\frac{p}{p_2} = \left[1 - \frac{(\gamma - 1)}{\gamma}\frac{(X - x)}{X}\right]^{2\gamma/\gamma - 1} \tag{2.36}$$

$$\frac{T}{T_2} = \left[1 - \frac{(\gamma - 1)}{\gamma}\frac{(X - x)}{X}\right]^{2} \tag{2.37}$$

Self-similar solutions to Equation 2.36 (and the analogous one from Equation 2.32, for flow velocity) have been developed and used to describe the flow fields behind unconfined detonations. An example of the variations

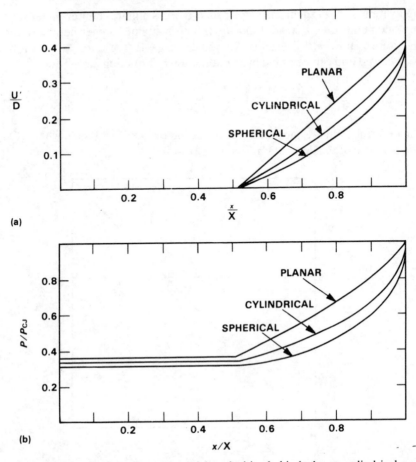

Figure 2.13   (a) Distributions of particle velocities behind planar, cylindrical and spherical C–J detonations; (b) distributions of pressure behind planar, cylindrical and spherical C–J detonations.

in flow velocity and pressure with non-dimensional distance, x/X for the flow behind planar, cylindrical and spherical detonations is shown in Fig. 2.13(a) and (b). It should be noted that the pressure gradients in the expansion depend only on the distance of the front from the detonation origin. As a consequence, the creation of further expansion fronts by lateral vents or openings, at the rear of a front propagating in a tube, has no influence on its properties, unless they operate in the vicinity of the subsonic reaction zone.

2.9 Concluding remarks

Section 2.1 emphasized that only a condensed account of available inform-ation on unidimensional theories was to be presented. In particular, detailed descriptions have only been given of those aspects which have been incorporated in treatments of real fronts. In this context, it is not unusual for a portion of a front, even interacting with a structure of complexly changing shape, to behave in a fashion analogous to that expected of a unidimensional detonation. The particular merit of unidimensional models is their accurate description of the average velocity of the leading front in mixtures well away from the limits of detonability. Consequently, they allow a reasonably adequate classification of the damaging potential of a detonation in various mixtures of this type. However, it is essential to appreciate their limitations.

Even for detonations in compositions well removed from the limits there are discrepancies of up to 15% between measured flow pressures and densities and those predicted by unidimensional theories. Again, such theories underestimate the thickness of reaction zones by factors of up to ten. For media approaching the limits of detonability, C–J theory overestimates the velocity of the leading front by 20% or more. The discrepancies between prediction and measurement of pressures and densities of the flow behind the front increase accordingly in such mixtures. Although the theory results in overestimates, caution is necessary in unreservedly applying it even to the design of the least complex of plant, such as a straight pipeline of constant cross-section. Thus, the predictions are essentially of average properties of the front. The description of real fronts in Chapter 3 emphasizes the importance of the variations occurring locally in velocity, pressure and density. Their local values can greatly exceed those predicted by unidimensional theories. Finally, it is only possible to appreciate the behaviour of detonations in plant of more complex shape by considering the structure of the front.

3

Structure of detonation fronts

3.1 General remarks

It has been standard practice to base safety considerations in the design of plant on the concept of a steady unidimensional detonation front. Again, methods of controlling and preventing detonations (to be described in Chapters 7 and 8) have a similar basis, despite the existence for some time of evidence for the non-steady and multidimensional nature of detonations. There are a number of reasons for this situation. For instance, comprehensive and easily applied theories have been developed for steady waves which result in tolerable descriptions of the average properties of the wave in readily detonable media in the absence of confinement or in the presence of straight containment walls of constant cross-section. As will become increasingly apparent, comprehensive theories for structured fronts are not available. Again, since the pressures developed in contained detonations are so high, approximate estimates of their magnitude may well suffice to demonstrate that preventative measurements are necessary. However, there are situations in which a knowledge of the structure of the front is essential. In particular, it is necessary in order to understand the interactions of a detonation with a change in confinement, to estimate local pressure histories and how these may be influenced by gradients and non-uniformities in the composition of the explosive medium, so that the maximum pressure likely to be generated may be estimated. Again, a knowledge of the structure of the front and how it varies with the properties of the medium may have applications to the investigation of explosions. Thus, the occurrence of characteristic tracks in dust deposits on tube walls may allow the identification of the origin of a detonation and characterize the composition and initial pressure of the mixture involved.

An example of the effects of the structure of a front on local pressure histories may serve to reinforce these arguments. Particularly pertinent is the work of Voitsekhovskii and co-workers [64] on detonations in mixtures of carbon monoxide, hydrogen and oxygen. They used the optical arrangement which is sketched in Fig. 3.1(a) with and without a schlieren system to record the 'unrolled' trajectories of the various shock fronts and surface of the cylindrical front. Figure 3.1(b) shows these, with continuous lines marking the shock fronts and hatched lines the reaction zones. BC is the transverse front and AA_2 the primary wave, with the perturbation AA_1 formed by the expansion of the products of reaction; corresponding pressure histories recorded along the wall at 12 different stations are shown below. The pressure scale is logarithmic, so that there is an approximate factor of three difference in amplitude of the pressure experienced at different positions. A similar factor exists in the time between the arrival of the leading front and the Taylor expansion fan. Such variations are typical of detonations encountered in mixtures close to their limits of detonability.

Even more complex distributions of pressure can occur. Figure 3.2 shows a sketch of a schlieren record of a front in a stoichiometric mixture of carbon monoxide and oxygen diluted with argon, in which a second triple point (and associated reaction zone) trails the first. The pressures in each region, calculated on the basis of the leading shock travelling at C–J velocity, 30% of the chemical energy liberated behind the first triple point and 70% behind the second are $19p_0$, $52p_0$ and $160p_0$ respectively. Thus, for this particularly complex form of detonation, local peak pressures may vary by a factor of as much as eight over approximately two pipe diameters. The implications of such wide variations and of the highly asymmetrical distribution of the fronts to the choice of an appropriate maximum pressure for calculating the response of a pipeline to such a detonation are obvious.

There is an extensive literature on the structure of detonations [14, 15]. Much of the experimental work therein has been performed with stoichiometric mixtures of fuel and oxygen, heavily diluted with argon to improve the regularity of soot track patterns. Important features of these studies (for instance the effect of increasing initial pressure of the medium in decreasing the spacing of transverse waves [65–67]) are discussed, particularly their application to fuel-lean mixtures with air, most likely to be produced by a malfunction of plant. Although the features emphasized are chosen for their practical import and are frequently empirical in nature, we have attempted to relate them to what is presently known of the fundamental processes involved. This should allow an appreciation of their application to the interaction of detonations with confinement (contained in Chapter 6) and to damage produced by detonations (in Chapter 7).

Since mixtures close to their limits of detonability are associated with waves with only a single transverse front, 'spinning' fronts are treated separately in Section 3.2. Following sections deal with experimental findings on multi-headed fronts and the gradual development of theoretical models describing them; Section 3.5 suggests safety matters to which the models should be applied.

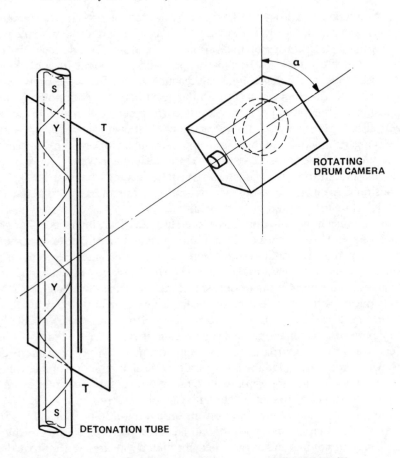

SS AXIAL SCREEN, BLOCKING RADIATION α = PITCH OF HELIX
TT OPTICAL SLIT   TRANSVERSED BY
YY TRAJECTORY OF DETONATION HEAD HEAD OF DETONATION

(a)

Figure 3.1 (a) Compensatory method for recording path of a spinning detonation wave; (b) unrolled spinning detonation front and pressure histories at 12 sites on the wall. (After Voitsekhovskii *et al.* [64].)

3.2 'Spinning' detonation fronts

The fact that stable spin is an intrinsic property of detonation waves in certain media confined in tubes of circular cross-section was recognized over fifty years ago. Following the original observations of the reproducible striations produced on high-speed photographic records of detonations in stoichiometric mixtures of carbon monoxide and oxygen [27, 68], Bone and co-

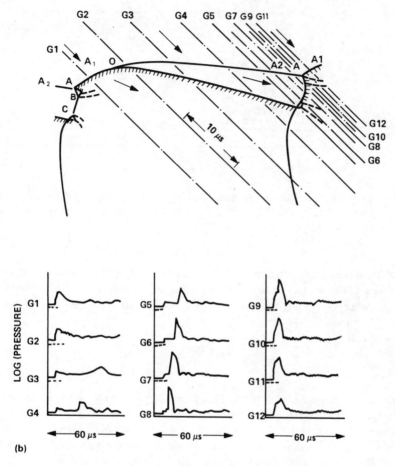

(b)

workers systematically investigated the phenomenon. They found it produced spiral cracking of glass tubes and etched a single helical track on the silvered surface of a tube [69–71]: they also found that neither the cross-section of the tube nor the insertion of a 1 mm ridge along the length of a 12 mm bore detonation tube had any effect on the phenomenon. Interestingly however, Bone *et al.* discovered that intense electrical fields did lead to irreproducible effects on both spin and the velocity of the wave. They concluded that spin was connected with the mode of coupling of the leading shock front and reaction zone. A fuller understanding of the mechanism of coupling of the shock and reaction zone arose later from theoretical studies [72–74], which showed that it occurred via an acoustic wave moving trans-versely across the main front propagating axially along the tube. By assuming

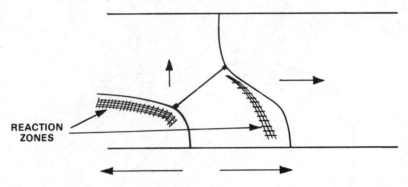

Figure 3.2 Asymmetrical stresses generated by a complex spinning detonation in a $CO-O_2-Ar$ mixture, in which 70% of the energy is liberated behind the second triple point (after Voitsekhovskii *et al.* [64]).

that the dimensionless acoustic impedance across the head of the front was infinite and the temperature ratio across the front was large, Fay [73] showed that the ratio of the pitch of the spin to the diameter of the tube p/d was given by:

$$p/d \simeq \frac{\pi(\gamma_0 + 1)}{\gamma_0 k_n} \qquad (3.1)$$

where γ_0 is the specific heat ratio of the products of the detonation and ranges from $\gamma_0 \simeq 1.2$ for undiluted mixtures of fuel and oxidant to 1.4 for fuel-lean mixtures of fuel with air. The constant k_n is a derivative of the Bessel function with a value of 1.841 for single-headed spin and increasing to 5.35 for four-headed spin. For a single-headed wave Equation 3.1 gives $p/d = 3.13$, close to the measured value of 3 [28]. Table 3.1 shows the close agreement obtained between the experimental measurements of pitch with the predictions from Equation 3.1 for tubes of different cross-section. In order to modify the results from Equation 3.1 to tubes of non-circular cross-section, values of modal number n and number of modes m were chosen to give closest agreement between theory and experiment. As the final columns of the table show, this was generally achieved for low values of n and m.

Although, as will be discussed in Section 3.3, the transverse waves are in fact weakish shock waves, experimental investigations of spin have confirmed the general applicability of acoustic theory in describing their properties [75–77]. However, later theoretical studies have shown that not all aspects of the process are understood. Thus, it has been shown theoretically that a perturbation in pressure, most probably produced by a partial reflection of leading front at the wall, will, in a reacting flow, rapidly intensify to form a transverse shock [78]. However, it is not possible positively to identify the mechanism whereby energy is dissipated to stabilize the strength of the front. Ideally, the mechanism should account for the experimental observation that fuel-lean mixtures favour low-frequency modes and more fuel-rich mixtures (where the thickness of reaction zone is generally very small compared with the diameter of the tube) favour the existence of multi-headed fronts [77]. It may be more profitable to extrapolate from conditions in the stabilized wave; then, for media with thin reaction zones, it is possible to envisage stabilization occurring via the prior reaction behind the Mach stem of the gas engulfed by

Table 3.1 Comparison of measured [69–71] and predicted [73] pitches of detonations in tubes of non-circular cross-section.

Section	Size (mm)	Pitch (mm)		n	m
		Measured	Calculated		
Square	12×12	41.0	43.3	0	1
Rectangle	9.8×12	42.0	43.3	0	1
	11×22	37.5	39.6	1	0
	13.5×22	72.8	79.4	0	1
	24×30	32.3	33.7	2	2
Equilateral	17	50.8	46.0	1	0
triangle	23	67–80	62.1	1	0

the transverse front. With single-headed spin the gas encompassed by the transverse wave will be compressed and heated by the decaying lead front to steadily decreasing pressures and temperatures. The resulting increased distance between reaction zone and transverse wave could well account for stability.

Information on the effects of composition of the mixture on spin is widely scattered throughout the literature. What is available is often conflicting and difficult to interpret. For instance, the results of an early study [79] of the effects of the initial pressure and composition of heavily-diluted mixtures of hydrogen and oxygen are shown in Fig. 3.3(a), (c) and (d) along with results for undiluted and fuel-rich hydrogen–oxygen mixtures (3.3(b)). They clearly illustrate that the generally-accepted phenomenon of single-headed spin for mixtures close to fuel-lean and fuel-rich mixtures is not influenced by the initial pressure of the mixture. This is in marked contrast with later results [80] for stoichiometric mixtures of hydrogen and oxygen, shown in Fig. 3.13, which indicate that the initial pressure of the mixture strongly influences the complexity of the structure of the detonation. As the hydrogen content of the mixture is increased, increasing the initial pressure of the diluted mixture leads to a change in structure. However, the effects of helium and argon on the complexity of the structure are puzzling. Defining the wavelength of spin as

48

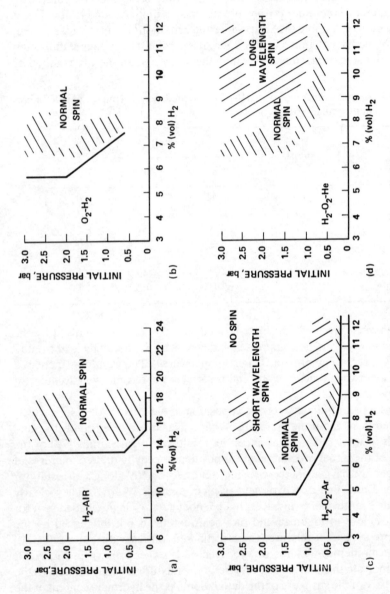

Figure 3.3 Influence of initial pressure and diluents on spin in oxyhydrogen detonations (after Gordon *et al.* [79]).

$\lambda = p/d$ Equation 3.1 can be rewritten in terms of the speed of sound in the burnt gas a_0 as

$$\lambda = p/d = \frac{\pi d}{a_0 k_n} \qquad (3.2)$$

Thus, the higher speed of sound in mixtures diluted with helium might be expected to lead to spin of short wavelength, not long wavelength as observed.

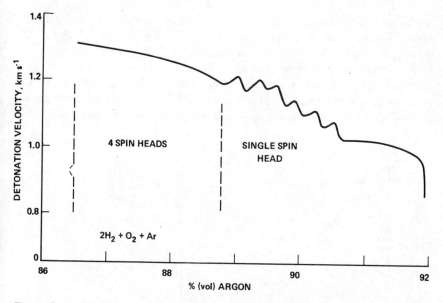

Figure 3.4 Influence of argon dilution of stoichiometric oxyhydrogen mixtures on wave velocity and spin-regime (after Munday *et al.* [81]).

Further confirmation of the effects of increasing the dilution of oxy-hydrogen mixtures in promoting single-headed spin comes from an elegant set of experiments in which the velocities of the front were measured using conventional ionization probes [81]. Figure 3.4 shows how increasing dilution by argon results in a progressive fall in the velocity of the wave, with failure occurring at a dilution of about 92% by volume of argon. Also shown are the effects of dilution on the nature of spin, with 4 transverse waves occurring between approximately 86 and 89% argon, changing to single-headed spin at ≥89% argon. The structures of the fronts were deduced from records from a ring of twelve ionization gauges on the circumference of the wall at a fixed distance from the origin of the detonation. The trajectories of the fronts are defined as oblique straight lines at an angle θ to a normal to the axis of the tube. From Equation 3.1 θ is given by

$$\arctan \theta = \frac{p}{\pi d} \tag{3.3}$$

and the velocity of the front along these trajectories v_t is given by

$$v_t = \frac{u_o}{\sin \theta} \tag{3.4}$$

where u_o is the detonation velocity along the axis of the tube, obtained from measurements such as those illustrated in Fig. 3.4. Figure 3.5 shows the development of the ionization histories from the 12 gauges for dilutions giving rise to single- and four-headed spin. The later portion of the ionization histories traces the trajectories of trailing ionization fronts. Incidentally, the distance of 19 mm between the crest and trough for single-headed spin allows an estimate of typical delays before the complete surface of a plate, normal to

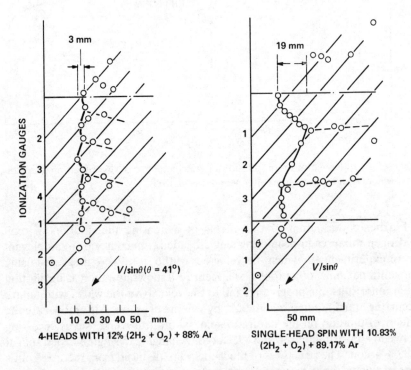

Figure 3.5 Effect of dilution on spin regimes, revealed by a ring of ionization probes (after Munday *et al.* [81]).

the axis of the tube, is subject to a reflected shock. Thus, with a velocity of 1.2 km s^{-1}, typical of marginally-detonable mixtures, the delay is about 15 μs.

Although the possibility of overshoot in pressure transducers must be borne in mind, it now seems well established that local pressure ratios in excess of those predicted by unidimensional theories occur in spinning fronts [14, 64, 82]. Indeed, it appears that the more complex the front, the higher the local pressure produced. For instance, it will be recalled that the calculated pressure ratio across a trailing triple point of the complex front occurring in mixtures of carbon monoxide and oxygen diluted with argon is as high as 160. Whether such complex waves occur generally or are influenced by the properties of the mixture and its confinement is not known, so basing analyses of maximum local pressures on their occurrence is probably not justified at present. A relatively simple analysis for a single triple point can be given in terms of the ignition of the medium, precompressed and heated by a C–J axial front, behind the transverse front [83]. Under such conditions the calculated pressure ratio across the transverse front is 126 for the diluted mixture of carbon monoxide and oxygen in which the experiments were carried out. The calculation assumes that the circumferential velocity of the front is the C–J value (obtained from standard computer programs) and the axial velocity of the front is (somewhat arbitrarily) 0.85 C–J.

3.3 'Galloping' fronts

'Galloping' fronts (in which regular oscillations occur in the velocity of the leading front as it propagates along a tube, with a frequency depending on both the potential energy release and the nature of any diluent present) have not received the attention they deserve, with experimental studies being confined to diluted mixtures of hydrogen and oxygen and of propane and oxygen [84–86]. There are two principal reasons for their potential importance. Firstly, they appear to be an extension of the phenomenon of spin, occurring in mixtures too close to the limits of detonability for a mechanism involving a single transverse front to retain its capability of continuously supporting a front. Thus, they are likely to occur in the mixtures produced by a malfunction of plant. Secondly, as is shown in Fig. 3.6(a), the regular peak velocities of the leading front can exceed the C–J velocity by as much as 35% with corresponding rises in local peaks in pressure [86]. Furthermore, the overdriven phase A persists over extended lengths of tube, say 0.1 m. Based on simple unidimensional theories of a planar and non-reactive shock, there can be a variation in the pressure ratio across the leading wave from 88 to 12 over a length of typically a metre.

Returning to Fig. 3.6(a), regions of (i) approximately constant velocity, (ii) slow acceleration and (iii) rapid acceleration have been investigated by a combination of schlieren photography and smoked-foil techniques. In region

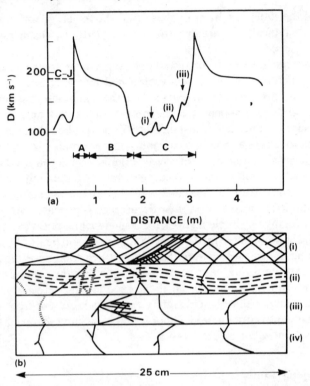

Figure 3.6 (a) Velocity versus distance record from microwave interferometry of a 'galloping' wave in $C_3H_8 + 5O_2 + 7.4Ar$, $p_0 = 50$ torr. (After Edwards and Morgan [87]). A 'galloping', B failure regime and C re-establishment; (b) Sketches of smoked-foil records, typical of 'galloping' waves, in $C_3H_8 + 5O_2 + 7.4Ar$, $p_0 = 50$ torr. (i) re-initiation approximately 5 cm from start; (ii) of slapping wave; (iii) attempt at re-establishment approximately 7 cm; (iv) slapping wave. (After Edwards and Morgan [86].)

(i) the flame and shock are separated by distances of at least 50 mm and no transverse front is present. In region (ii) oblique shocks start to occur and apparently promote rapid acceleration (iii). The overdriven regime is apparently a result of the classical Urtiew and Oppenheim [87] 'explosion within an explosion' process, described in detail in Section 5.2.

Sketches of smoked foils illustrating the main features of the decay and re-establishment of the wave are shown in Fig. 3.6(b). Record (i) exhibits re-initiation occurring some 5 cm from the start of the trace, resulting in a strong blast front moving forwards and a retonation wave moving backwards. The initially overdriven front is characterized by a large number of trajectories of triple points which decrease to form a regular pattern from 15 to 25 cm. Record (ii) is of the 'slapping' wave in the narrower dimension of the tube and some scouring of the soot deposit, probably by a detached section of the reaction zone, is visible. In (iii) and (iv) the 'slapping' wave and an attempt at re-initiation at about 7 cm (iii) are visible.

Obviously much more data are needed on for instance, the likely effects of air (rather than oxygen) as the oxidizing medium, of the initial pressure and temperature of the mixture and of the absence of confinement on the frequency of oscillations and on the ratio of maximum to minimum velocities. However, the grave experimental difficulties in obtaining such data must be recognized – for instance, the experimental studies must be carried out in straight tubes of some tens of metres in length, on account of the long wavelength of the oscillations and the absence of information on how the phenomenon is likely to be influenced by bends in the experimental tube. Such information is not likely to be available in the immediate future: however, the very existence of such a phenomenon in near-limit mixtures emphasizes the dangers of underestimating peak pressures in design studies by using simple unidimensional models of detonation waves.

3.4 Experimental studies of multi-headed fronts

Detonations in mixtures well away from detonability limits are multi-dimensional. Detailed information on structures is contained in a number of reviews [14, 15, 88]. Careful experiments by Strehlow and co-workers [65–67] on soot-track records inscribed in various mixtures of fuels with oxygen, in the presence and absence of diluents, have revealed the existence of different types of wave. Firstly, there are equilibrium fronts, the time-average properties of which are constant and the structure of which repeats regularly. An example of an equilibrium front is a spinning wave. Secondly, there are time-average steady fronts without the regularity of repetitive structure. Typical examples of these are detonations in stoichiometric mixtures of simple molecules of fuel and oxygen, heavily diluted by a noble gas such as argon. The increased temperature in the flow behind shock fronts of the same velocity, resulting from the high specific heat ratio of argon, enhances the regularity of the structure. Finally, there are truly transient fronts. Typically these are associated both with fuels which are resistant to detonation (such as methane) and with more readily detonable hydrocarbons of high molecular weight in mixtures which are close to the limits of detonability [89]. The experimental difficulties of studying transient waves are obvious, consequently most available data come from experiments on time-average steady fronts. Furthermore, much of the work has been carried out in tubes of rectangular cross-section, in order to suppress the effects of transverse fronts in the narrower walls. The effects of the interactions of the transverse fronts travelling in orthogonal directions are by no means clear.

It is now recognized that spin is the limiting case of the multi-dimensionality of structure of fronts. Thus a number of transverse waves run orthogonally across the leading wave, reflecting from one another and any containment walls. The surface of the leading front consists of a series of bulges (the Mach stems, behind which are located reaction zones) and a series of depressions which are essentially decaying blast waves [90–92]. Further reaction zones are located in the flows behind the transverse waves. Figure 3.7(a) shows a section of such a front, with reaction zones denoted by hatched lines and unreacted media by dots [32]. The Mach stems are lettered OM, the transverse waves with associated reaction zones OT and the acoustic tails of these waves TR. The directions of motion of the various fronts are shown by arrows. Figure 3.7(b) is a sketch of a typical detonation cell etched on a deposit of dust on the walls of a channel by the triple points. Patterns composed of such cells, with the dimensions S_c and L_c depending on the fuel molecule, the initial pressure and the composition of the explosive media, but typically with $S_c \simeq 0.6 L_c$, are produced by planar, cylindrically-expanding fronts [35] on the confining walls and on a flat-plate over which a spherically-expanding detonation travels [93]. There have been no systematic attempts to characterize the structure of detonations in either self-decomposing or two-phase media. However, since structure is apparently a direct outcome of the fundamental mechanisms governing the propagation of a detonation, there is no reason to doubt its presence in such media.

In order to conceive the three-dimensional structure of the front, it has been suggested envisaging the confining walls as being packed with an equivalent number of octahedrons and tetrahedrons of cross-section related to S_c and in which a combination of spherical and cylindrical waves converge and diverge repeatedly [92]. The picture becomes very complex when the ratio of dimensions of a rectangular tube is not an integer, in which case the orthogonal systems of waves move relative to each other to produce a pattern which repeats every few cycles.

Figure 3.7(c) shows how the velocity of the leading front, as revealed for instance by streak schlieren photography, varies along the length of the cell. The factor by which the velocity of the leading front (following the collision of the Mach stems) exceeds the C–J velocity (D_{CJ}) varies, depending on how close the medium is to its limits of detonability. It can be as high as 1.5 for marginally detonable media, but for mixtures well away from their limits it is 1.2–1.3 [94]. The velocity falls with distance to the C–J level at one-third to one-half the length of cell with a further decrease to a terminal velocity of about $0.8 D_{CJ}$ for readily detonable media and $0.6 D_{CJ}$ for marginally detonable media.

Experimental measurements of the velocity of transverse waves close to the triple point in readily detonable media indicate that they are weak waves with Mach numbers, M_t, $1.1 < M_t < 1.2$ [82, 88]. Thus, there is some justification for treating them as acoustic waves in analyses of their spacing, as in Section 3.5. Furthermore, they suffer little or no attenuation throughout the length of the cell [91]. The velocity of transverse waves in media approaching their

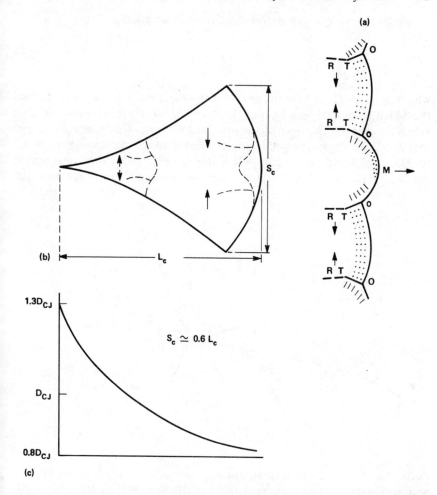

Figure 3.7 Instantaneous profile of a multi-dimensional front (a), detonation cell etched on a deposit on tube wall (b), and corresponding axial velocity of the leading front within the cell (c). OT, transverse front; TR, trailing acoustic wave; OM, Mach stem; O, triple point; ||||, reaction zone; :::, unreacted medium.

limits increases to approach the limiting value of 1.84 M_{CJ} for a detonation with single-headed spin (Equation 3.2). The strength Z_t of the transverse front in a coordinate system rendering the triple point O stationary (Fig. 3.8) can be defined [95] as

$$Z_t = \frac{p_3 - p_1}{p_1} = \frac{p_3}{p_1} - 1 \qquad (3.5)$$

or, since the pressures across the slipstream OS are equal,

$$Z_t = \frac{p_2}{p_1} - 1 \tag{3.6}$$

where p_3, p_2 and p_1 are the pressures behind the transverse wave OT, behind the Mach stem OM and behind the decaying wave OI, respectively. For stoichiometric oxyhydrogen mixtures diluted with argon, it has been observed that $Z_t \simeq 0.5$ for mixtures well removed from the limits, increasing to $Z_t = 1.3$ for marginally detonable media [88]. Consequently, the increased strength of the transverse waves in the latter media can more than compensate the

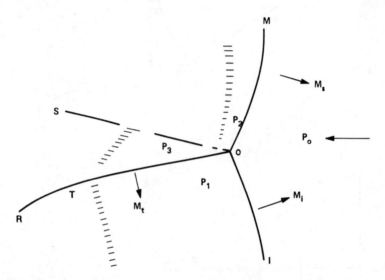

Figure 3.8 Weak transverse wave structure for readily-detonable media in a co-ordinate system rendering triple point stationary (after Strehlow and Biller [95]). OM, Mach stem; OI, decaying leading shock; OS, slipstream; OT, transverse shock; ||||, reaction zones.

amplitude of local pressures for the decreased axial velocity of the leading fronts. Further details of the properties of transverse fronts are contained in Section 6.3, describing experimental studies of the interaction of detonation waves with wedges.

An assessment of the response of a structure to a detonation requires a knowledge of local variations in pressure with time. Thus, information on the disposition of reaction zones and their associated Taylor expansion waves is required. However, it should be borne in mind that with truly multi-dimensional fronts there is no reason to expect the existence of a well-defined sonic plane, as predicated in idealized C–J detonations. Surprisingly, there

Table 3.2   Hydrodynamic thickness x_h of detonation waves in various mixtures [96].

	$2H_2 + O_2$	$2H_2 + O_2 + 3Ar$	$C_2H_2 + 2.5O_2$	$C_2H_2 + 2.5O_2 + 10.5Ar$
Initial pressure (torr)	530	610	230	610
x_h (mm)	8.32	6.84	7.00	7.5
L_c (mm)	2.4	1.9	0.7	1.5
x_h/L_c	3.8	3.6	10	5

have been only two systematic experimental investigations of the locations of
expansion regimes [96, 97]. In the first of these a fragile detonation tube was
used to trace the propagation of the rarefaction wave produced on its rupture,
to locate where the flow became supersonic [96]. Table 3.2 gives results for the
hydrodynamic thickness of the front in terms of cell lengths for a number of
mixtures at just below atmospheric pressure. It is commonplace to extrapolate from these to suggest that $\leq 10L_c$ separates the leading front and the
reaction zones. It has been suggested, with some justification, that the decay
in strength of transverse waves in the flow behind the leading front can be used
to give some indication of the location of the surfaces at which sonic flow first
occurs. Figure 3.9 shows results for $2H_2 + O_2$ and $3C_2H_2 + 7O_2$ mixtures,

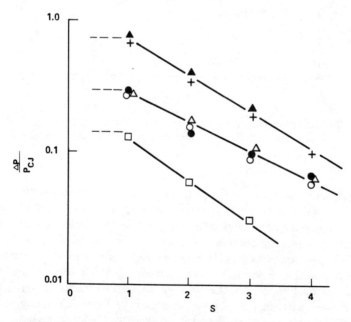

Figure 3.9   Decay of non-dimensional pressure of transverse waves with distance
$\Delta 2H_2 + O_2$ at 100 torr; ▲, +, ●, ○, □, $3C_2H_2 + 7O_2$ at various pressures (after
Edwards *et al.* [97]).

suggesting that the waves decay in 2 to 4 L_c, in reasonable agreement with the results in Table 3.2 [97]. Figure 3.10 is a time-resolved record of pressure in a $2C_2H_2 + 7O_2$ mixture. It shows clearly the fall in strength of the transverse front in the later stages. Note that the rate of decay after about 40 μs agrees closely with that predicted in an ideal isentropic expansion.

Thus, from a knowledge of the dimensions of a detonation cell it is possible to estimate approximately the duration of the peak pressures generated by a detonation. The relationship between L_c and S_c varies with the initial pressure of the mixture, falling from $L_c/S_c \sim 2$ for pressures of 0.1 bar to 1.3–1.4 at an

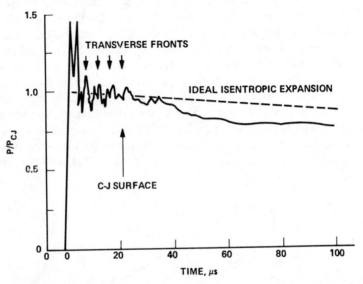

Figure 3.10 Experimental determination of decay in pressure behind a detonation in $2C_2H_2 + 7O_2$ compared with decay in an ideal isentropic expansion (after Edwards *et al.* [97]).

initial pressure of 1 bar [98]. Unfortunately, experimental data on the dimensions of detonation cells and how they vary with the nature of the fuel molecule, composition and initial pressure of the detonable medium are not as extensive as might be wished. The soot-tracks recorded for mixtures of oxygen with hydrogen, acetylene, ethylene and methane in the presence and absence of additives have been noted previously [66, 67]. More recently and of more practical import are the observations of soot tracks for mixtures of different fuels with air [98]. These are shown in Table 3.3, along with an estimate of the index of dependence of cell length on the initial pressure of the mixture. Generally, the cell length is approximately inversely proportional to the initial pressure of the mixture.

Table 3.3 Cell lengths of detonations in stoichiometric mixtures of various fuels with air, oxygen and nitrogen at an initial pressure of 1 bar and dependence of L_c on initial pressure [98].

Gas mixture	L_c (mm)		$n = \dfrac{\log L_c}{\log p_0}$
	Measured	*Extrapolated*	
H_2 + Air	15.9 ± 2	—	—
H_2 + $0.5O_2$	—	0.6	−1.35
CH_4 + Air	—	500 ± 80	—
CH_4 + $2O_2$	4.5	—	−1.21
C_2H_2 + Air	13.6 ± 1.6	—	−0.88
C_2H_2 + $2.5O_2$	0.3	—	−0.91
C_2H_4 + Air	39 ± 6	—	−0.50
C_2H_4 + $3O_2$	—	1.0	−0.65
C_2H_6 + Air	88 ± 14	—	−0.79
C_2H_6 + $3.5O_2$ + $10.5N_2$	—	52	—
C_2H_6 + $3.5O_2$ + $7N_2$	—	15	−0.86
C_2H_6 + $3.5O_2$ + $3.5N_2$	—	7.1	−0.91
C_2H_6 + $3.5O_2$	—	1.2	−1.07
C_3H_8 + Air	72 ± 12	—	−0.44
nC_4H_{10} + Air	—	85	—

In general it appears that the more resistant the fuel molecule is to detonation, the larger are the dimensions of the cell. Section 3.5 gives some advice on semi-empirical methods for estimating dimensions of cells from shock-tube measurements of an induction period for the onset of exothermic reaction. These deserve careful consideration in the case of mixtures on which, for various reasons, no other information is readily available. For instance, the size of cells in detonation-resistant fuels is so large that direct measurement is usually impractical, and the patterns produced by such fuels are generally highly irregular. Additional difficulties in the interpretation of soot tracks can arise from the presence of slapping waves and the existence of irregular finer structure which has yet to be satisfactorily explained. Arguably, the area in which least information is available is the effect of stoichiometry of fuel–oxidant mixtures on the dimensions of cells. That the spacing of transverse waves on detonations in fuel-lean mixtures of ethylene and air is very strongly dependent on the composition of the mixture is demonstrated by the curve in Fig. 3.11 [99]. The line represents the best fit to a compilation of various workers' experimental results for mixtures of ethylene and air, probably the most intensively studied system.

Since the dimensions of the detonation cell depend on the initial pressure, degree of dilution and stoichiometry of the explosive media and the chemical

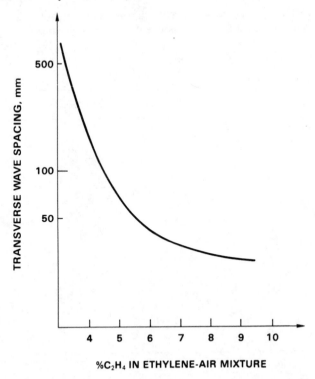

Figure 3.11 Compilation of experimental measurements of spacing of transverse fronts on detonations in mixtures of ethylene with air of different composition. (After Moen *et al.* [99].)

properties of the fuel, there is some danger of oversimplification in offering advice on the duration of peak pressures. However, for mixtures of fuel and oxygen, initially at about atmospheric pressure and not too far from stoichiometry, spacing of transverse fronts is typically in the range 1–10 mm. For stoichiometric mixtures in air this increases by a further factor of ten. There could well be a further magnification factor of about ten for mixtures approaching the fuel-lean limit. Thus there are likely to be wide divergences in the shape of pressure histories in the fuel-lean mixtures with air, which may be encountered in an accident in chemical plant, from those generally observed in experimental studies on undiluted stoichiometric mixtures of fuel with oxygen. Taking a distance of $5S_c$ for the decay of the wave and assuming the average axial velocity of the front to be C–J, which will approach 3 km s^{-1} for stoichiometric mixtures of fuel with oxygen, typical durations of maximum pressures are in the range 1–10 μs. The mean velocity of the leading wave in mixtures with air is reduced by a factor of about two, so that the arrival of the expansion front in mixtures close to stoichiometric is delayed by between 5 and 50 μs after the arrival of the leading front. Provided that the relationship between the dimensions of the cell and the hydrodynamic thickness of the shock is independent of the stoichiometry of the mixture, the duration of high pressure can approach 500 μs. Consequently, some caution is required when applying the results of experimental studies of damage caused by detonations (which have been invariably carried out with stoichiometric mixtures) to predictions of the effects of a detonation in a fuel-lean mixture with air. In addition to the existence of highly-localized peak pressures in the latter mixtures, the increased thickness of the wave may well result in a pressure-type rather than an impulsive loading of the structure. Although there have been no systematic studies of dimensions of cells and thicknesses of fronts in two-phase and self-decomposing media, the induction zones are generally larger than for homogeneous mixtures of fuel and oxidant. Thus, similar considerations should apply to their potentially damaging effects.

3.5 Theoretical treatments of multi-headed fronts

It is possible to produce an approximate estimate of the spacing of transverse waves using a modified ZND model to estimate the delay period τ behind the Mach stem components of the leading front. Taking average properties of the flow behind the Mach stems, the induction period can be transformed into a length of induction zone which, in turn, can be empirically related to the length of the detonation cell. It will be recalled that the ZND model involves defining τ in an Arrhenius form by $\ln \tau = \rho_m{}^a \exp(E/RT)$, where ρ_m is the initial density of the medium, a is the index describing the dependence on density $(-1 < a < -0.5)$, E is the global temperature coefficient of the reaction steps leading up to the exothermic recombination processes and T the temperature of the flow behind the Mach stem. In order to utilize readily obtainable shock tube data on E and a, it is necessary to consider what is the appropriate temperature to characterize the flow regime behind the attenuating Mach stems. For detonations in marginal media the experimental evidence suggests that an appropriate mean temperature lies between the values in the flow behind $1.5M_{CJ}$ and M_{CJ} fronts, and for readily detonable media between the values for $1.3M_{CJ}$ and M_{CJ} fronts.

At this stage some cautionary remarks are in order. Measurements of the temperature dependence of induction periods, taken at temperatures well below those corresponding to flows behind M_{CJ} shocks, are frequently extrapolated to the higher temperatures behind the Mach stems of a detonation wave. It is quite common for there to be significant changes in temperature coefficient of a global reaction scheme over an extended temperature range. Again, shock tube experiments are frequently carried out with mixtures which are heavily diluted with argon to minimize the thermal effects of pre-flame reactions. Argon is likely to be an inefficient collision partner in the steps initiating the exothermic reactions and its effectiveness not strongly influenced by temperature. However, detonable media formed by the release of flammable gases or vapours into air are likely to contain significant concentrations of water vapour and carbon dioxide, both of which are likely to be much more efficient third bodies in the initiating steps than argon and could well cause significant changes in temperature coefficients at temperatures behind the Mach stems of detonation fronts, where both carbon dioxide and water will be rapidly decomposed.

The sparse experimental data available on the dimensions of detonation cells necessarily result in the frequent application of readily-available induction periods obtained, either from experiments in shock tubes or from theoretical analyses based on a postulated reaction scheme [100–103]. Again, the later method frequently involves extrapolating widely from the temperature range over which the temperature dependence of the rate constants of the individual reaction steps have been measured. The length of the induction zone L_i is defined as either

$$L_i = \tau_i \bar{M}_s a_0 (\rho_0 / \bar{\rho}_1) \tag{3.7}$$

or

$$L_i = \tau_i (\bar{D} - \bar{u}_1) \tag{3.8}$$

where a_0 is the speed of sound in the unreacted medium, $\bar{M}_s a_0 = \bar{D}$ is the average velocity of the Mach stem, $\bar{\rho}_1 / \rho_0$ the average density ratio across the Mach stem and $\bar{u}_1$ the average velocity of flow behind the front. Assuming that previous results for the relationship between L_i and L_c can be extrapolated over a range of initial pressures, compositions and fuels:

$$50 \, L_i \leq L_c \leq 100 \, L_i \tag{3.9}$$

Figure 3.12 shows Westbrook's [100] results for the effects of composition, expressed as equivalence ratio (ratio of fuel to oxidant in the mixture divided by ratio of fuel to oxidant in stoichiometric mixture), on the length of induction zone for various hydrocarbons in mixtures of fuel and air, presumably at an initial pressure of 1 bar. Note that the behaviour of fuel-lean mixtures of all the fuels closely models that of ethylene, with the rapid increase in L_i (and thus spacing) occurring at low concentratons of fuel, as previously noted. An elaborate reaction scheme involving 87 individual reaction steps was used to model the kinetics of the processes involved in the induction period. Table 3.4 gives a comparison of cell lengths predicted for stoichiometric mixtures in oxygen and air with the measurements in Table 5.3. Allowing for the limited comparison and the possibility of errors in the kinetic data on which the predictions are based, $L_c = 50 \, L_i$ seems appropriate for hydrocarbon fuels mixed with oxygen. For mixtures with air a smaller magnification factor, say 15, gives reasonable agreement, except for acetylene. The general agreement between measured values of L_c and that deduced from the semi-empirical correction of the theoretical predictions lends some confidence to the use of authenticated kinetic schemes for

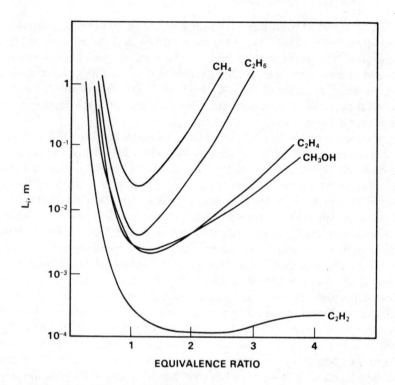

Figure 3.12 Influence of stoichiometry of fuel–air mixtures on predicted length of induction zone (after Westbrook [100].)

Table 3.4 Comparison of predicted and experimental values of cell lengths for stoichiometric mixtures of hydrocarbon with oxygen and air [100].

Fuel–oxidant mixture	Calculated cell length (mm)	Measured cell length (mm)
$CH_4 + 2O_2$	7.5–15	4.5
$CH_4 + Air$	1500–3000	500 ± 80
$C_2H_2 + 2.5O_2$	0.3–0.6	0.3
$C_2H_2 + Air$	15–30	13.6 ± 1.6
$C_2H_6 + 3.5O_2$	2.5–5.0	1.2
$C_2H_6 + Air$	250–500	88 ± 14
$C_2H_4 + 3O_2$	1.5–3.0	1.0
$C_2H_4 + Air$	100–200	39 ± 6

predicting the effect of stoichiometry on the dimensions of cells. It should be noted however, that the C–J velocity was used to deduce the effective average temperature behind the leading front – the possibility of higher velocities in fuel-lean mixtures may well modify the predictions. Further confirmation of the general applicability of the $2 L_c \leq x_h \leq 10 L_c$ criterion comes from their successful application in describing the diffraction of a detonation at an abrupt expansion in area.

A significant proportion of the chemical energy driving the front (say $\geq 25\%$) is released behind the transverse waves [94, 104]. Thus, an analogous treatment of induction zones behind the transverse fronts would add considerable confidence to an extrapolation of available data to different systems. However, there are a number of reasons for doubting whether this can be accomplished, amongst which are the possibilities of pre-flame reactions conditioning the gas in the flow behind the blast wave portions of the leading front. It should be noted that this is an important feature in the ignition delays of knock-prone hydrocarbons ignited by a combination of planar incident and reflected shocks [105]. Again, molecules engulfed by different portions of the blast fronts will be heated and compressed to significantly different temperatures and pressures for different times before they enter the transverse fronts. It is highly unlikely that the use of an average speed of sound and particle velocity will produce a satisfactory description of so complex a flow field. However, the degradation of the tail of the transverse wave into an acoustic front, together with the quenching of the reaction zone can readily be appreciated. The tails of these are engulfing gas compressed and heated to low pressures and temperatures.

To date, the most complete theory describing the spacing of transverse fronts has only found application in predicting the effects of argon dilution and initial pressure on spacing in stoichiometric mixtures of hydrogen and oxygen. The theory is complex and requires a knowledge of accurate chemical kinetic data for the complete reaction scheme, including the recombination steps which are the principal source of energy release. Whilst global kinetic data for the initiation steps occurring during the induction period are available (or can be calculated) for a wide range of mixtures of hydrocarbons and oxidants [100], the same is not true of the recombination steps. Nevertheless the merits of the theory in describing the effect of the initial pressure of the mixture and the velocity of the leading front on spacing deserve attention. Following early theoretical studies of the amplification of acoustic perturbations in exothermically reacting media [106–109], Barthel [80, 110] developed a method of describing the propagation of acoustic waves in the flow field behind the leading shock of a unidimensional detonation front. His calculations showed that an acoustic front in such a flow field became convoluted and he interpreted the spacing of transverse waves in terms of the distance between the caustics produced by convolution. Figure 3.13 is a comparison of the predictions from the theory for $2H_2 + O_2 + ZAr$ mixtures with experimental

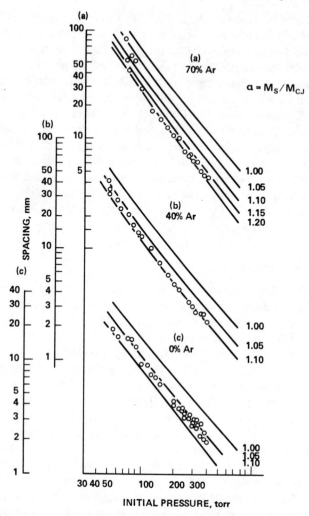

Figure 3.13 Comparison of predicted (full lines) and experimental measurements (open circles) of spacing of transverse fraction in $2H_2 + O_2 + ZAr$ mixtures (after Barthel [80].)

measurements of spacing. The theory performs well both in describing the effects of initial pressure of the mixture and of the degree of dilution (Z) on the spacing of transverse waves. As might be expected from the observed variations of the leading front in a cell, the degree of overdrive $\alpha = M_s/M_{CJ}$ required for the closest agreement between theory and experiment lies in the range $1.2 \leq \alpha \leq 1.05$, with the requisite value of α decreasing with decreasing dilution of the mixture.

Some simplifications to Barthel's [110] model are possible. These have resulted in a treatment which has potentially a much wider range of applicability and suggests that the spacing of transverse fronts is relatively insensitive to the distribution of energy released in the reaction zone [111]. This reduces the required input to the model to the lengths of induction and reaction zones and specific heat ratio of the products of the detonation. For media with reaction zones much thinner than induction lengths, as occurs at initial pressures approaching 1 bar, further simplification is possible, and predictions based on this relatively simple model describe the effects on spacing of initial pressure, degree of overdrive and dilution by argon of stoichiometric oxyhydrogen mixture, although underestimating the actual value of spacing by a factor of about ten. It is perhaps surprising in view of the reasonable adequacy of the simplest of the models that it has not found more widespread application.

3.6 Concluding remarks

Before rehearsing the implications of the structure of a detonation front to its potential for causing damage, a brief apology for the continued use of C–J concepts in a chapter on structured fronts may be appropriate. Partly, this is a continuation of generally accepted practice, involving the advantages of applying the readily available data from which C–J velocities can be calculated simply. Again, it will be recalled that the C–J velocity corresponds closely with the average axial velocity of the leading front within a detonation cell and thus provides a tolerable description of the global properties of multi-headed detonation waves from which the bulk of experimental data have been obtained. However, there are compelling arguments for a proper consideration of the correction factors to be applied to unidimensional theories, to account for the effects of the multi-dimensional nature of detonations, when analysing the response of containment. For instance, the effects of the structure of fronts become steadily more pronounced in the fuel-lean mixtures most likely to be encountered following a malfunction in plant. It is also reasonable to infer that similar considerations apply to self-decomposing fuels in the absence of oxidants, with the largest corrections to predictions based on unidimensional theories being required in media at pressures just above the critical level.

It is convenient at this stage to recapitulate on the departures from those predicted by unidimensional theory of the properties of detonation fronts in marginally detonable media. Some of these will be discussed in greater detail in Chapter 6. Here, we examine the magnitude of the variation in the maximum local pressure in the absence of any change in confinement.

We have noted a number of mechanisms whereby the local pressures produced by the complex structures of real detonations can greatly exceed those predicted by unidimensional theory. Notable amongst these are the phases in galloping detonations, during which the leading front propagates at a velocity well in excess of the C–J value. Another example is the enhancement in pressure produced in the reaction zone behind a second triple point, which has been observed to occur with spinning waves in certain media. With detonations in marginally-detonable media smoked-foil records reveal patches of fine structure [98], resulting from attempts by a failing wave to re-establish itself. Whilst Barthel's model [110] indicates that increasing fineness of structure is associated with an increase in the strength of the leading front, it is difficult to estimate accurately cell sizes in the patches of fine writing and thus difficult to estimate the pressures occurring there. Again, there is no known way of predicting the probable locations of these regimes of re-establishment – indeed, it is likely that the process is stochastic. Too little is known of the effects of the medium and confinement on all these phenomena to be able to make more than tentative suggestions about their occurrence and likely magnitude. However, it is worth noting that it is unlikely that more than two of these mechanisms can exist simultaneously in a particular medium confined by straight walls of constant cross-section. For instance, high pressures can be generated in the re-ignition zones of a galloping wave, as well as in the phase in which the leading front propagates at well above C–J velocity. Fortunately however, the re-ignition zone is one which has been compressed and heated by a front much weaker than the standard C–J front, so that the maximum pressure generated should not exceed that obtained in the following treatment, i.e. two to three times the C–J level. Indeed, it is unlikely that any of the processes presently described would result in the factor by which the local pressure exceeds the C–J value being more than three.

Since the pressure of the mixture treated by the leading Mach stem in a single detonation cell is equal to that in the mixture heated by an adjacent decaying front and the associated transverse wave, it is possible to base a simple analysis on the known variations of the leading front within the cell. Recalling the relationship between the strength of a non-reactive and planar shock front and its Mach number from Chapter 2:

$$\frac{p_2}{p_1} = \frac{2\gamma M_s^2 - (\gamma - 1)}{(\gamma + 1)} \tag{2.7}$$

and that at the origin of a detonation cell in a fuel-lean mixture near its limits $M_s/M_{CJ} = 1.5$ with $\gamma = 1.4$, the local pressure there can be over twice that calculated for a C–J wave. With less marginal mixtures $M_s/M_{CJ} = 1.3$, so that the ratio of maximum to C–J pressure falls to less than two. The lowest local pressure observed to occur at the end of the cell in cells in marginally-detonable mixtures corresponds with M_s/M_{CJ} having fallen to about 0.6 i.e. to about one-third of the C–J value, emphasizing the wide variation which can occur locally.

We are unaware of any systematic studies of abnormally high pressures behind detonations in two-phase media. However, the likely increase in hydrodynamic thickness, resulting from generally longer ignition delays with particles or droplets, indicates that the occurrence of high-pressure zones associated with re-establishment may feature more frequently than in homogeneous media.

4

Detonable media

4.1 General remarks

It is worth emphasizing at an early stage the severe difficulties encountered in an attempt to produce a comprehensive list of detonable media. For instance, the potential hazards are often only recognized after an explosion in a plant and in many such instances it has been impossible to pronounce unambiguously that the damage resulted from a detonation. Furthermore, at the elevated pressures and temperatures normally associated with processing plant, the relationship between the original mixture and that which exploded is often by no means clear. In this context, the possibility of the formation of compounds, such as peroxides and hydroperoxides in cool flames in mixtures of hydrocarbons with oxygen and which are readily decomposable to form radicals, may be of particular importance in modifying limits of detonability. Thus, whilst every attempt has been made here to produce an exhaustive list of detonable media, there will undoubtedly be a number of omissions, especially of media in which small concentrations of active species are present.

The experimental difficulties in producing large volumes of gaseous mixtures of uniform composition, together with the requirement for energetic initiators, have meant that only a limited number of studies have been carried out on detonability of partly and completely unconfined media. It is necessary to consider how best to extrapolate from information on confined detonations, so Section 4.2 discusses the role of confinement in the initiation of a detonation.

Whilst the hazards of mixtures of fuel and oxidant are widely appreciated, there are a number of gases and vapours which can, on their own, support a detonation. Notable amongst these, on account of their widespread use, are acetylene and ozone. These and other examples are discussed in Section 4.3, and the increase in pressure limit by some two to three orders of magnitude compared with that in the presence of an oxidant, in the case of acetylene, is noted.

It is frequently necessary to deduce limits of detonability from known or calculated values of flammability. A case in point is mixtures of two or more fuels with an oxidant. Section 4.4 lists available comparative data on limits for confined and unconfined detonations and flammability limits for mixtures of both fuel and air and fuel and oxygen. Neither limits of flammability nor of detonability, however, are absolute quantities, they depend on the technique of measurement. For flames there are small but detectable differences in the limits for upward and downward propagation. Detonability limits are also affected by direction of propagation and by tube diameter, initiator characteristics, wall effects etc. Measurements must be applied with caution.

There are evident requirements for methods of prediction of detonability limits and techniques for extrapolating from known values for simple molecular structures to those for more complex, but related, molecules. One method of predicting limits from the effects of composition on the distance required to form a detonation [112] is described in detail in Chapter 5. An alternative procedure, based on experimental measurements of the decrease in detonation velocity occurring as the diameter of a pipeline is reduced, has been suggested [26]. However, too little experimental information is available and the gathering of the missing data is likely to be as onerous as measuring the limits for the method to be of general usefulness. Thus, Section 4.5 selects a method which has been applied to mixtures of alkanes and alkenes with oxygen [113]. Following sections describe the limited experimental data on detonations in mixtures of fuel with an oxidant other than oxygen, and the effects of diluents, initial pressure and temperature on detonability.

It is possible to produce a detonation in the initial absence of a preformed fog or suspension of dust. For instance, the strong blast wave produced by an energetic igniter can result in flows of sufficient velocity to scour a liquid or dust deposit on the walls of a pipeline and thus produce a flammable suspension [114]. Such a process is particularly important in the case of explosions in mine galleries [115]. Section 4.9 considers the detonability of clouds of dusts and droplet mists and the features which distinguish them from detonations in homogeneous mixtures of gases.

4.2 Confined and unconfined detonations

Not only have confined detonations been studied more widely than unconfined detonations, they are the type most likely to occur in practice. This is on account of one of the two principal, but partly conflicting, effects of the walls. The first is their potential in generating turbulence in the flow ahead of the flame to promote the transition from a deflagration to a detonation; thus, a flame in a detonable mixture contained in a pipeline can readily accelerate to approach sonic velocity, when a shock is formed in the mixture ahead of the flame. The initial velocity of such a flame is a function of the product of the laminar burning velocity (S_u), typically $S_u \sim 1$ m s^{-1}, and the expansion ratio (ϵ = ratio of the density of the reactants to that of the products), typically

$5 \leq \epsilon \leq 12$. The acceleration of the flame from these modest velocities occurs via a combination of the turbulence generated by the flame itself and that produced in the flow of unreacted mixture. These result in an increase in the area of the flame through its surface wrinkling and a transition to turbulent burning, the velocity of which is approximately an order of magnitude higher than the laminar burning velocity. The combined effects result in the formation of a shock ahead of the flame, possibly within 50 or 60 tube diameters, and the final transition to detonation in a length of up to 100 tube diameters.

Although wall-generated turbulence promotes the early stages of the initiation of a detonation, there is evidence that it can reduce the velocity of an established front. This is particularly evident with detonations in tubes in which uniformly-spaced protuberances, in height a tenth or less of the tube diameter, are introduced, as for instance in the well-known example of helices of wire, commonly referred to as Shchelkin spirals. These are particularly effective in reducing the distance required for the production of a detonation wave of uniform velocity. However, they can reduce the experimental velocities to much below the theoretical values for a unidimensional front. Thus, detonation velocities in mixtures well away from the limits of detonability contained in smooth-walled tubes, which we have seen are accurately predicted by C–J theory (Equations 2.16 and 2.17), can be reduced to velocities as low as half the C–J velocity in tubes with regular arrays of obstructions [116] (Fig. 4.1). This suggests that up to three-quarters of the

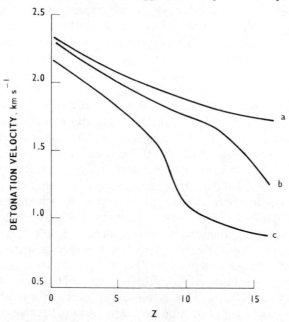

Figure 4.1 Detonation velocities in mixtures of $C_3H_8 + 5O_2 + ZN_2$ in the presence and absence of Shchelkin spirals. (a) smooth walls; (b) Shchelkin spiral, pitch 20 mm; (c) Shchelkin spiral, pitch 4 mm [116].

chemical energy can be dissipated by wall-generated turbulence. Thus, peak internal pressures produced by detonations in pipelines with corrugated walls should be significantly lower than those in smooth-walled versions. This is not to suggest that the introduction of roughened walls is a recommended procedure for ameliorating the effects of detonation; rather, the possible effects of pronounced roughness of walls should be kept in mind when investigating incidents where the damage is less than might be expected from C–J wave.

Cylindrically-expanding waves can be produced in partially-confined situations. For instance, consider an explosive medium confined between two flat and parallel plates, with initiation from a source bridging the gap between them. The voltage required to break down the gap between the plates will depend on the composition and initial pressure of the explosive medium and the width between the plates. For typical compositions and initial pressures of 1 bar, the breakdown voltage will be about 1 kV mm^{-1}. Thus, the extremely high voltages required to break down gaps of widths characteristic of those likely to occur in chemical plant (≥ 100 kV) suggest that cylindrically-expanding waves will rarely occur in practice. Situations in which they may occur involve the generation of a lightning-like discharge. A possible example is the cleaning by water jets of non-inerted tanks in a bulk-oil carrier, where static voltages built up from charges on droplets can result in a lightning-type discharge; similar conditions might occur in a land-based storage tank during cleaning operations. Initiation by linear explosive charges or flames has a very low probability. Consequently, cylindrically-expanding detonations rarely occur in practice. Partly because of their rarity and partly because initially-cylindrical waves will tend to adopt spherical symmetry beyond the limits of the confinement, cylindrically-expanding fronts have not been studied in any great detail.

The growing realization that large-scale escapes of flammable vapours are not uncommon events on a worldwide scale, and that widespread damage may be produced by the explosion of the resultant unconfined cloud of vapour [117] has instigated a wealth of studies on the initiation of spherical detonation fronts. Thus, following the classical study of Zel'dovich and co-workers [118], noteworthy later examples are given in references [119] to [133] inclusive. Many of these have been involved in attempts to establish the limits of detonability of fuels in air, particularly fuels such as methane which do not form readily detonable mixtures even in confined situations. In order to minimize the energy required to initiate spherical waves with such fuels, the experiments have frequently been performed with varying degrees of dilution of the mixture with nitrogen (Fuel + YO_2 + ZN_2) and the results extrapolated to the nitrogen content of air. Nevertheless, much of the experimental work described in these references has involved the use of very energetic sources, such as large charges of condensed explosives. Again, because of the severe experimental difficulties associated with producing large volumes of mixtures of homogeneous composition, some form of containment, for example a large plastic balloon, has often been employed. The possibility of reflection of pressure waves from such containers or from the ground, together with the use of powerful igniters means that the confidence limits which can be placed on limits of detonability and wave velocities for spherical detonations are wider than those for confined detonations.

Arguably the uncertainties are minimized for the results obtained following the free expansion of a planar detonation front through a sudden and large change in area, with the same mixture on either side of the nozzle [3, 118]. Providing the inlet is of a diameter greater than a critical value, determined by the properties of the explosive medium, a hemispherically-expanding detonation is produced downstream of the nozzle. With any walls parallel to the axis on the expansion side of the nozzle, at a sufficient distance for reflections from them not to arrive back at the axis of symmetry until the detonation has propagated over ten or more critical diameters, reliable measurements of limits and radial velocities of the front are obtained.

At this stage it is worth noting that the concept of spherical propagation implies a considerable degree of idealization when applied to accidental releases of vapour. It involves either the total absence of local inhomogeneities in the cloud or their presence in sufficiently small pockets for them to result in only minor perturbations in the local velocity of the front. Again, there are constraints on the initiating source. It should be either a point source or a spherical one. If the latter, the energy must be deposited uniformly over the surface in order to prevent local asphericities in the wave close to the source. While experimentalists make strenuous efforts to achieve the conditions necessary for spherical propagation, these are frequently unavailing in the early stages of the detonation. Thus, it is important to bear in mind possible asymmetries in the development of a large-scale detonation.

4.3 Gases and vapours which are detonable in the absence of an oxidant

The potential hazards associated with the possibility of a detonation developing in homogeneous mixtures of fuel and oxidant are widely recognized. However, there are a number of gases and vapours which decompose exothermically at sufficiently high rates to support a detonation in the absence of an oxidant. The monograph of Stull [12] and the handbook of Bretherick [134] cite a number of such compounds. The explosive potential of many of these has only been recognized following an accident, because of the expense and labour involved in conducting experimental studies of detonations to cover the range of operating conditions likely to be experienced in plant. Thus, it is unlikely that existing lists of detonable gases and vapours are exhaustive.

Probably the most important detonable gases and vapours in the context of amounts produced and transported are gaseous acetylene [135–138], ethylene at pressures in excess of 7 MN m^{-2} [12], ozone [139] and hydrogen peroxide vapour [140]. Of these, the problems involved in producing, transporting and utilizing acetylene in chemical synthesis have received most attention [135, 141]. Detonation waves and some of their properties, such as the velocity of the front and pressure limits in hydrogen azide (HN_3) [142, 143], chlorine azide (ClN_3) [142, 144], possibly bromine azide (BrN_3) [145], chlorine dioxide [146] and nitric oxide [147] have been studied. Other gases and vapours which are detonable in certain circumstances are diazomethane [148], ethylene oxide [149–153] but not propylene oxide [152], possibly butadiene [154–156], cyanogen [12, 134], propargyl bromide [12, 134], vinyl acetylene [134] and, possibly, hydrides of boron [134]. There are common features in the thermal decomposition of derivatives of acetylene, such as diacetylene [157, 158], so that a range of alkyne derivatives may be detonable. Consequently, the possibility of a detonation should be seriously considered for all compounds which decompose exothermically. However, it is worth noting that there are no recorded well-authenticated examples of detonations in self-decomposing media occurring in the absence of confinement.

Table 4.1 Experimental data on detonation properties of exothermically-decomposing vapours.

Fuel	Detonation velocity in tube of infinite diameter $(km\, s^{-1})$	Pressure to which D_∞ applies $(N\, m^{-2})$	Pressure limit $(N\, m^{-2})$
100% C_2H_2	1.92	8.1×10^5	$\sim 1.5 \times 10^{5*}$
90% H_2O_2 + 10% O_2	1.82	$<2.7 \times 10^4$	$2 \times 10^3 < p_e < 2.7 \times 10^3$
100% HN_3	2.60	6.7×10^2	$\sim 1.3 \times 10^2$
100% ClN_3	2.30	2.0×10^3	<7
92.3% O_3 + 7.7% O_2	1.82	2.13×10^4	$\sim 1.3 \times 10^3$

* There is some evidence suggesting that the pressure limit may be lower when powerful initiators are used. The corresponding detonation velocity may well also be lower in this case.

Table 4.1 lists experimental values of detonation velocities, corrected for losses to the wall (D_∞) and the initial pressures at which the measurements were made. Included in Table 4.1 are the experimental data on the pressure limit for sustainable detonations with the various self-decomposing fuels (p_e). It is interesting to note the similarities in the properties of detonations in ozone and hydrogen peroxide, whereas there are considerable differences in the apparently more closely chemically related compounds, HN_3 and ClN_3. Finally, the implications for the fuel-rich composition limit of mixtures of self-decomposing fuels and an oxidant should be noted. Provided that the initial pressure of the fuel is above the pressure limit, there is the possibility of a smooth transition from detonations driven by oxidation to detonations driven by the decomposition of the fuel with increasing concentration of the fuel. Consequently, a fuel-rich limit may not exist. The analogous situation may well occur with the fuel-lean limit, when ozone or hydrogen peroxide vapour is the oxidant.

4.4 Comparison of detonation limits for confined and unconfined detonations with flammability limits for mixtures of hydrocarbons with oxygen and air

Flames can be produced in a wide variety of fuels other than hydrocarbons. Zabetakis [159] gives a fairly comprehensive list of flammability limits together with information on minimum temperatures for autoignition of mixtures of these with air. However, there have been few studies of confined detonations in mixtures containing fuels other than hydrocarbons. Notable exceptions are ammonia [160, 161], cyanogen [162–164] carbon disulphide [19] and tetramethylsilane [165]. Information on spherical detonations is even more limited, with Carlson's work on a comparison of the limits of a number of hydrocarbons mixed with oxygen the only readily-available source [166]. Even this is open to potential criticism, in that the experiments were carried out in a small spherical bomb of diameter ~30 cm. Consequently, there is a possibility that the effects of the initiator were still present, resulting in the production of overdriven fronts. In this context, it is probably worth emphasizing the onerousness of determining unconfined limits. Large volumes of mixtures of uniform composition are required in order to ensure that effects of the initiating source and of inhomogeneities in composition are absent. For instance, it is advisable to measure limits of spherical detonations of readily-detonable mixtures in confinements of at least 1 m in diameter. For less readily-detonable mixtures or fuels such as methane, this figure should ideally be increased by a factor of five to ten.

On account of these difficulties, recourse is frequently made to known flammability limits in estimating probable detonation limits of fuels for which no other information is available, or for mixtures with two or more fuels present. Such a procedure will usually result in a safe overestimate of the range of detonable compositions; however, the cautionary comments previously made on the possible extension of the upper limit self-decomposing fuels must be borne in mind. Again, there is some evidence that the flammability range for self-decomposition flames in acetylene is narrower than the detonable range [41].

Table 4.2 is a compilation of the most recent data on flammability and detonation limits for fuels for which some directly comparable information exists [167]. It includes measurements of limits for both confined and unconfined detonations for mixtures of the fuels both with oxygen and air though again these quantities depend on the technique of measurement, see Section 4.1. Considering first the flammability limits, obvious discrepancies

Table 4.2 Detonation limits (vol. %) for confined and unconfined explosions and flammability limits (vol. %) [167].

Fuel	Confined detonation limit, O_2		Confined detonation limit, air		Unconfined detonation limit, O_2		Unconfined detonation limit, air		Flammability limit, air		Flammability limit, O_2	
	Lower	Upper	Lower	Upper	Lower	Upper	Lower	Upper	Lower	Upper	Lower	Upper
C_2H_6	3.60	46.4	2.87	12.20	11.0	39.0	4.0	9.2	3.0	12.4	3.0	66.0
C_3H_8	2.50	42.5	2.57	7.37	7.0	31.0	3.0	7.0	2.1	9.5		
nC_4H_{10}	2.05	38.0	1.98	6.18			2.5	5.2	1.8	8.4		
nC_8H_{18}	1.55	17.3	1.45	2.85					0.95			
C_2H_4	4.10	60.0	3.32	14.70	9.2	51.0	3.5	8.5	2.7	36.0	2.9	80.0
C_3H_6	2.50	50.0	3.55	10.40	6.7	37.0			2.4	11.0	2.1	53.0
C_2H_2	2.90	88.8	4.20	50.0	6.7	68.0			2.5	80.0		
$CH_3C{\equiv}CH$					5.7	49.0			1.7			
MAPP $(37.8\%^{*}\,CH_3C{\equiv}CH)$							2.9	10.1				
Petrol†			~5.6	~9.4								
CH_3OH	9.50	64.5	5.1	9.8					6.7	36.0		
C_2H_5OH									3.3	19.0		
$C_2H_5OC_2H_5$	2.6	>40	2.8	4.5	4.7	29.0			1.9	36.0	2.0	82.0
Cyclo C_3H_6									2.4	10.4	2.5	60.0
Cyclo C_6H_{12}	1.4	29.0			6.7	39.0			0.57	7.8		
C_6H_6	1.55	36.0	1.60	5.55					1.3	7.9		
Xylene	1.05	26.5							1.1	6.4		
CH_3COCH_3	3.3	40.0							2.6	13.0		
CH_3CHO					13.0	48.0			4.0	60.0		
H_2	15.0	90.0	18.3	58.9					4.0	75.0	4.0	95.0

* MAPP 37.8% $CH_3C{\equiv}CH$, 26.1% $CH_2{=}C{=}CH_2$, 18% C_3H_6, 10% $n-C_4H_{10}$, 7.4% C_2H_6
† Mass basis

exist in published data. There has been a historical trend for the generally accepted limits to widen. Typical examples in Table 4.2 are the lower limits for propane and ethylene both in air and oxygen. As might be expected, there is little change in the lower limit when air is replaced by oxygen (see, for instance, the figures for the alkane series of hydrocarbons). However, the upper limit is dramatically extended for mixtures with oxygen. In general, the results for detonation limits reflect those for flammable limits, but the range of detonable compositions is narrower than the flammability limits of each fuel listed, both for mixtures with oxygen and with air. Again, the limits of unconfined detonations are narrower than those for confined detonations. Although there are only small changes in the lower limit for confined detonations when oxygen is replaced by air, the lower limit for spherical detonations is increased by a factor of about two for mixtures with oxygen. This is compensated for by the much higher upper limit, a factor of three or more, for spherical detonations in mixtures with oxygen. However, some caution must be exercised in extrapolating these factors to other fuels. They may well partly reflect the use or more powerful initiating sources with air mixtures, so that the comparison of lower limits is probably more suspect.

Figures 4.2 and 4.3 represent some of the results given in Table 4.2 in a manner which may be more helpful as a guideline to detonable limits for hydrocarbons on which no information is available. Figure 4.2 for confined and Fig. 4.3 for unconfined detonations show the ratios of fuel to air and fuel to oxygen of detonable mixtures, plotted against the corresponding ratio of mixtures stoichiometric with respect to steam and carbon dioxide as products, ϕ_{st}. The vertical lines represent the range of detonable mixtures for each fuel, the sloping dashed lines represent reasonably conservative estimates of upper and lower limits of detonable compositions. The equations for detonations in tubes of the lines shown are, for the lower, ϕ_l, and upper, ϕ_u,

$$\log \phi_l = 1.08 \log \phi_{st} - 0.84 \tag{4.1}$$

$$\log \phi_u = 1.06 \log \phi_{st} + 0.64 \tag{4.2}$$

for mixtures with oxygen and

$$\log \phi_l = 0.60 \log \phi_{st} - 0.78 \tag{4.3}$$

$$\log \phi_u = 1.13 \log \phi_{st} - 0.56 \tag{4.4}$$

for mixtures with air. The less extensive results for the limits of spherical detonations are tolerably well represented by only two lines, representing lower and upper limits in mixtures with both air and oxygen. Perhaps fortuitously, lower and upper limits for spherical detonations expressed in terms of stoichiometry are not very different from those for confined mixtures

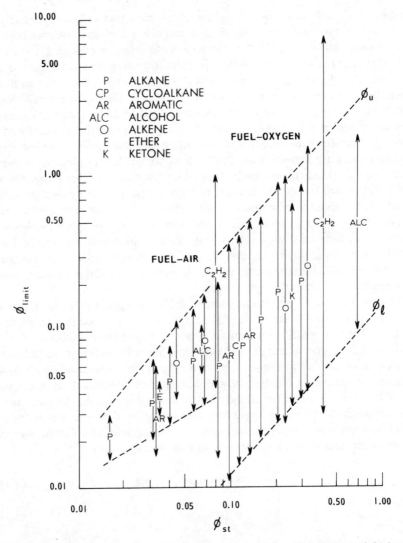

Figure 4.2 Composition limits for confined detonations in mixtures of fuel and oxygen and fuel and air.

of fuel and air. The relevant equations are

$$\log \phi_l = 0.51 \log \phi_{st} - 0.81 \tag{4.5}$$

$$\log \phi_u = 1.17 \log \phi_{st} + 0.60 \tag{4.6}$$

It should be noted that the upper limit for acetylene, predictably, is considerably higher than that given by the equations for both confined and unconfined situations. Interestingly, the lower limit for acetylene is also

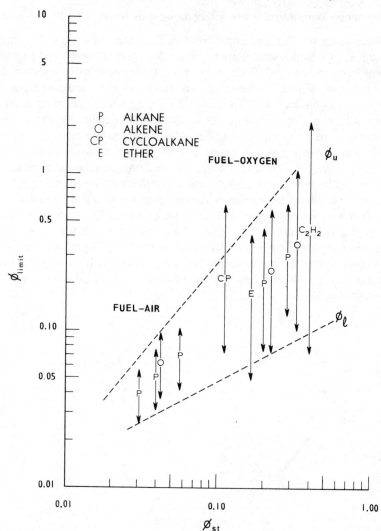

Figure 4.3 Composition limits for unconfined detonations in mixtures of fuel and oxygen and fuel and air.

anomalously lower than the prediction. Again, the upper limit for a spherical detonation, in the single example of the cycloalkanes, is higher than the empirical equation indicates. There do not appear to be any suggestions in the literature that pure cyclohydrocarbons are detonable. A possible explanation is that the blast wave from a strong initiator results in partial conversion of less thermally stable hydrocarbons into products such as acetylene.

4.5 Homology hypothesis for predicting detonation limits

It has been suggested that the upper limit for detonations in mixtures of fuel and oxygen approaches stoichiometricity with respect to steam and carbon monoxide as products, ϕ_s, as the fuel molecule becomes more resistant to detonation [168]. Figure 4.4 illustrates this effect for spherical detonations in mixtures of various fuels with oxygen, with the minimum initiating energy representing the resistance to detonation of the fuel molecule. An alternative explanation is that the upper limit for detonations in mixtures of hydrocarbons and oxygen arises because of the energy associated with the formation of soot [113, 165]. However, a more formal approach, capable of predicting both lower and upper limits, is evidently desirable. Such a treatment for confined detonations in various hydrocarbons in the presence of oxygen involves the assumption that the parent hydrocarbon rapidly breaks down in the shock-compressed region (preceding the reaction zone), to produce similar products from similar initial ratios of $C:H:O$, no matter what the structure of the original molecule [113]. For instance, homology defines an alkane C_nH_{2n+2} as equivalent to $nCH_2 + H_2$, and an alkene C_nH_{2n} as equivalent to nCH_2.

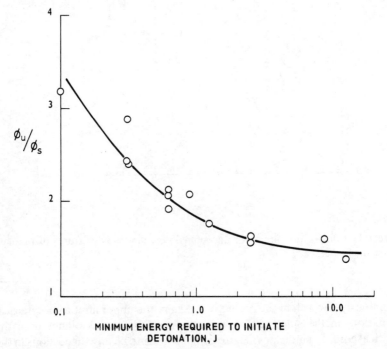

Figure 4.4 Approach of upper limit for spherical detonations to stoichiometry, with respect to CO and H_2O as products, as fuel molecule becomes increasingly resistant to detonation [168].

Table 4.3 Experimental results for homology of lower and upper limits for confined detonations in mixtures of fuel and oxygen [113].

Fuel	Lower limit		Upper limit	
	% Fuel	% Homology	% Fuel	% Homology
CH_4	8.25	15.2	55.8	71.6
C_2H_6	3.60	10.1	46.4	72.2
C_3H_8	2.50	9.3	42.5	74.7
nC_4H_{10}	2.05	9.3	37.95	75.4
nC_5H_{12}	1.50	8.4	33.0	74.7
C_2H_4	4.1	7.88	41.2	74.0
C_3H_6	2.5	7.14	50.0	75.0

Table 4.3 lists the original experimental results for confined mixtures of alkanes and alkenes with oxygen on which the hypothesis is based. It indicates that the maximum upper limit for confined detonations in mixture of alkanes and alkenes with oxygen is not likely to exceed a percentage homology of 75.4%. The average value for the upper limit is 74%. Extrapolation from the results for the fuel-lean limit is more problematical, there being an apparent downward trend in homology with increasing molecular weight and with alkenes having lower values than alkanes.

For convenience the lower limits for unconfined detonations in mixtures of oxygen and fuels not listed in previous tables are given in Table 4.4. The results are from a variety of sources and, since the limit is likely to be influenced by the initial pressure of the mixture and the dimensions and shape

Table 4.4 Experimental measurements of lower limits for confined detonations in mixtures of fuel and oxygen

Fuel	ϕ_l (mole %)	Fuel	ϕ_l (mole %)	Fuel	ϕ_l (mole %)
CH_3Cl	10.1	$C_{10}H_{16}$	0.9	CO	40.0
CH_2Cl_2	11.0	$C_6(CH_3)_6$	0.55	O_3	9.0
$CHCl_3$	18.0				
$C_2H_2Cl_2$	6.6	CH_3OH	9.5		
C_2Cl_4	12.5				
		$C_4H_4O^*$	2.6	NH_3	25.0
$C_{10}H_{22}$	0.7				
$C_{16}H_{34}$	0.46	$Si(CH_3)_4$	1.8	H_2	15.5
$C_{10}H_{18}$	0.7			C_2N_2	36.7

* Furan

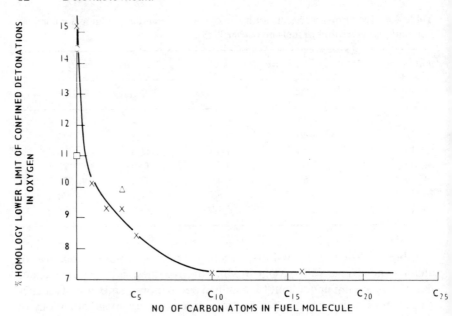

Figure 4.5 'Homology' hypothesis of lower limits in confined mixtures of fuel and oxygen [113]. ×, alkane; ○, CH_3Cl; □, CH_2Cl_2; △, $Si(CH_3)_4$.

of the cross-section of the detonation tube, a rigorous comparison is inappropriate. Figure 4.5 shows the results for lower limits of oxygen mixtures (expressed in terms of homology for alkanes), halogenated hydrocarbons and tetramethylsilane plotted against the number of carbon atoms in the fuel molecule. It suggests that, for molecules with more than five carbon atoms, the lower limit approaches a homology limit of just over 7%.

4.6 Detonations with oxidants other than oxygen

Although there is a wide range of oxidants in the form of gases and vapours, capable of producing flammable mixtures with a variety of fuels, there is only limited information on detonations in such mixtures. Amongst such oxidants are halogens, ozone, hydrogen peroxide vapour, oxides of nitrogen and chlorine dioxide. The most intensively-studied system is that of hydrogen and chlorine; measured detonation velocities in confined stoichiometric mixtures are $D_c = 1.73$ km s^{-1} [169] and for spherically-expanding fronts, $D_u = 1.47$ km s^{-1} [170], which is considerably lower than the C–J velocity of 1.68 km s^{-1}. Levin and co-workers give some information on how the minimum energy required to initiate a spherical detonation in stoichiometric mixtures varies with the initial pressure [171]. Detonation velocities and formation distances for confined detonations in mixtures of hydrogen and nitrous oxide have been measured, and a fall in the lower limit observed when the initial pressure of the mixture was increased [172]. Anomalously high pressures have been measured close to the position at which a detonation first forms in confined mixtures of ammonia and oxides of nitrogen. Again, it is worth recapitulating that pure gaseous nitric oxide at pressures in excess of 1 bar has been shown to be capable of supporting detonations with velocities of at least 2.1 km s^{-1} [147], so that anomalies are likely to occur in fuel-lean mixtures with hydrocarbons. However, there are no reports of systematic studies of pressure and composition limits for any of the oxidants listed. Thus, in order to estimate detonation limits, recourse to available data on flammability limits is necessary.

Table 4.5 Comparison of flammability limits of selected fuels with various oxidants [159, 173].

Fuel	Lower limit (mole % fuel)				Upper limit (mole % fuel)			
	O_2	Cl_2	N_2O	NO	O_2	Cl_2	N_2O	NO
H_2	4.0	4.1	3.0	6.6	95	89	84	66
NH_3	15.0		2.2		79		72	
CH_4	5.1	5.6			60	70		
C_2H_6	3.0	6.1			66	58		
C_2H_4	2.9		1.9		80		40	
C_3H_6	2.1		1.4		53		29	

Publications by Zabetakis [159] and Coward and Jones [173] list flammability limits for a restricted range of fuels in a number of oxidizing media. Table 4.5 gives a comparison of flammability limits for some simple fuel molecules in oxygen with those in chlorine, nitrous and nitric oxides. In general, the limits are narrower for fuels mixed with the latter oxidizing agents than when they are mixed with oxygen. Little, if anything, is known about the influence of diluents on flammability limits with the less common oxidizing agents. Consequently, it is necessary for designers faced with the problems associated with such mixtures to arrange for experimental measurements of either flammability or detonation limits.

4.7 Influence of initial pressure and temperature on detonability

Although there have been a number of investigations of the relationship between the velocity of confined detonation waves and the initial pressure and temperature of the medium (to be described in Chapter 5), there is little direct information on their effects on detonability. What is available comes mainly from studies of the effect of initial pressure of self-decomposing fuels on the minimum diameter of the pipeline through which a detonation will propagate [135, 142–144]. Figure 4.6 illustrates a compilation of the results of a number of studies of pure acetylene [174]. For initial pressures lying above the line detonations are possible in long enough pipelines: at lower pressures the explosive wave propagates as a deflagration, no matter what the length of pipeline. Guidelines of this type were used in the design of German plant during the 1939–1945 war to manufacture acetylene which was the feedstock for the production of various organic chemicals [46]. They proved their value in the industry's record of safe performance.

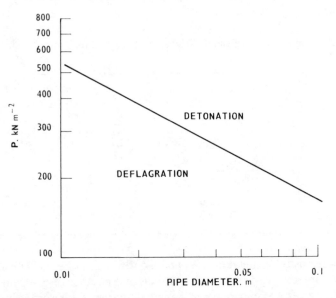

Figure 4.6   Influence of initial pressure on the critical diameter of pipe required for detonations in pure acetylene (after Sargent [174]).

There have been no systematic studies of the effect of initial temperature of gases such as acetylene on its detonability. It is worth noting that rates of decomposition of acetylene [175] and hydrogen and chlorine azides [176] are high in the presence of metallic surfaces at temperatures of $\geq 250\,°C$. Thus, any studies of detonability carried out at temperatures much above $100\,°C$ are likely to be of limits related to a mixture of thermally unstable gas and the products of its decomposition.

Similar considerations apply to the influence of initial temperature on the limits of detonability of confined mixtures of fuel and oxidant. Autoignition temperatures of alkanes in air decrease with increasing molecular weight from $540\,°C$ for methane to approach $200\,°C$ for *n*-nonane, and can be as low as

175 °C for aldehydes, nitrates and ethers [159]. The autoignition temperature for carbon disulphide is as low as 90 °C. Thus, for most fuels, it is only possible to carry out experiments on the effects of temperature over a very limited range. A particularly pertinent observation on this score comes from the comparison of the transition to detonation behind reflected shock waves in mixtures of *n*-octane and air with that in mixtures of iso-octane and air [105]. The transition was found to occur much more readily with the 'knock-prone' hydrocarbon, *n*-octane, because of the conditioning of the mixture in the flow behind the incident shock, in which various chemically-excited species are produced from the parent hydrocarbon.

Available information is therefore confined to a limited range of temperatures [177]. However, a temperature rise of 50° results in a narrowing of the limits of mixtures of hydrogen and oxygen at initial pressures ≥ 1 bar, with the fuel-lean limit occurring at higher partial pressures of hydrogen and the fuel-rich limit at lower partial pressures. However, the limited results for mixtures of methane and oxygen at 25 bar indicate a widening of the limits at the higher temperature. Although there are obvious dangers in extrapolating from such limited data, it is interesting that the results do not appear to correlate with the expected effects of temperature and pressure on burning velocity. Thus, burning velocities generally increase with increasing temperature of the mixture, and mixtures (such as hydrogen–oxygen) with high burning velocities at atmospheric pressure generally exhibit more pronounced increases in burning velocities at enhanced pressures than do those with lower burning velocities (such as methane–oxygen).

It is again difficult to generalize from the scant data available on the effects of initial pressure on the limits of mixtures of fuel and oxidant. Results from the same source [177] suggest that the upper limit for mixtures of hydrogen and oxygen tends towards higher partial pressures of hydrogen, as the initial pressure of the mixture increases from 1 to 25 bar. There appears to be little change in the lower limit of mixtures of these gases over the same range of pressure. Both lower and upper limits of mixtures of methane and oxygen appear to be independent of the initial pressure over the range 1 to 10 bar. Table 4.6 lists experimental results for the detonable limits of mixtures of hydrogen and nitrous oxide at pressures ≥ 1 bar. Also included for comparative purposes are the limits of mixtures of hydrogen and air at 1 bar. With nitrous oxide as the oxidant, the lower limit falls with increasing pressure to approach that of mixtures of hydrogen and air at 1 bar. Pressure has apparently no effect on the upper limit.

In terms of practical applications, it is unfortunate that our understanding of the likely effects of pressure on detonability is limited to confined mixtures of fuel and oxidant in the main at sub-atmospheric pressures. The data come from studies of the effect of initial pressure of the mixture on the spacing of transverse wave fronts [65–67], which were described in detail in Chapter 3. In summary, the effect of increasing the pressure of the mixture is to increase the

Table 4.6   Influence of Pressure on Limits for Confined Detonations [172].

Mixture	Initial pressure 1 bar		Initial pressure ≤ 10 bar	
	Lower limit (% H_2)	Upper limit (% H_2)	Lower limit (% H_2)	Upper limit (% H_2)
H_2–N_2O	25	60	20	60
H_2–air	19.3	58.9		

available chemical energy and consequently to decrease the spacing of the transverse waves, so broadening the limits of detonability.

In view of the inconsistencies in the data, it seems advisable to appeal to information on flammability limits for fuels which have not been studied, for mixtures of fuels, for unconfined media and for pressure greater than 1 bar. In general, increasing the initial pressure and temperature of the mixture leads to an extension of flammability limits, with a more dramatic increase of the fuel-rich limits.

4.8 Influence of additives on detonability

The effect of nitrogen as a diluent on mixtures of fuel and oxidant has been discussed in a comparison of composition limits for confined and unconfined detonations in mixtures of fuel and oxygen with those for mixtures of fuel and air (Section 4.3). The narrowing of limits, principally via a reduction in the upper limit, observed in experiments with air is a common feature of most additives. A study of detonations in confined mixtures of hydrogen and oxygen showed that additions of nitrogen, argon, water vapour and iodo-methane reduced the limits [178]. A tentative explanation of this is that a reduction in the temperature of the leading front leads to an increase in the induction period for formation of the flame, which is sufficiently large to result in the separation of shock and reaction zones. Addition of fuels such as benzene and furan (capable of sustaining detonations in oxygen themselves) were found to produce results which are difficult to interpret – additions of benzene had little effect on the limits and the complex effects of furan may be partly explicable in terms of the observation that a condensed polymer, $C_{45}H_4O$, could be formed. Later studies of confined mixtures of tetramethyl-silane and oxygen indicated that the upper limit may be related with energy losses to freshly-formed surfaces in the deposition of silicon dioxide [165], in analogy with the formation of soot controlling the upper limit of detonations in mixtures of fuel and oxygen [133].

In general, all the mechanisms involved in the action of additives are still far from being fully understood. For instance, confined mixtures of either hydrogen and oxygen or deuterium and oxygen, diluted to near the limits with hydrogen, oxygen, deuterium or carbon dioxide are characterized by regimes of detonations of low velocity [179]. These are apparently connected with changes in the reaction scheme which lead to the formation of significant amounts of either hydrogen peroxide or deuterium peroxide. Similar experiments on stoichiometric mixtures of hydrogen and oxygen and of deuterium and oxygen, diluted with argon or helium, have shown that the mixtures with

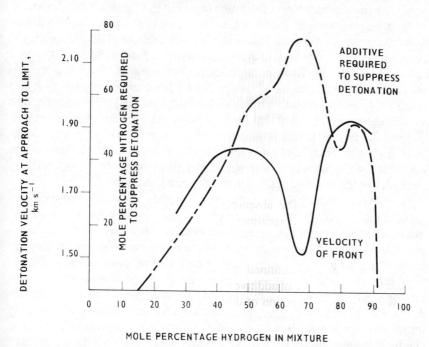

Figure 4.7 Amount of nitrogen required to suppress confined detonations in H_2–O_2 mixtures, together with the velocity of the front at the approach to the limit (after Miles *et al*. [178]).

hydrogen have wider limits than those with deuterium [180]. The reasons for this have not been resolved.

Figure 4.7 gives some indication of the large amounts of nitrogen required to suppress detonations in confined mixtures of hydrogen and oxygen [178]. Included in the illustration is the complex curve representing how the velocity of the detonation varies with the amount of hydrogen in the mixture. The second peak in the curve (at high concentrations of hydrogen) can be accounted for by the high speed of sound in hydrogen. Intuitively, it might be expected that the lowest amounts of additives would be required to suppress detonations in mixtures producing the lowest detonation velocities. However, the opposite is the case. An addition of 80% nitrogen is required for mixtures containing just under 70% hydrogen in which the detonation velocity is just over 1.5 km s^{-1}. At present, the only safe inference which may be drawn is that the amount of additive required falls sharply as the composition of the mixture approaches the lower and upper limits.

In summary, great caution must be exercised in any consideration of the use of additives to inhibit detonations, and it is advisable for their efficiency to be tested experimentally. Although small quantities of a wide range of halogenated hydrocarbons have been found to inhibit the flammability of mixtures of fuels and oxidants by modifying the chemical reactions, including explosions of suspensions of coal dust in air [181] and the rate of decomposition of acetylene [175], it would be dangerous to assume that similar additions will suppress initially overdriven detonations. For instance, the experimental observation that additions of halogenated hydrocarbons to coal particles suspended in oxygen had no influence on their ignition [182], indicates that such inhibitors may be ineffective in preventing detonations in heterogeneous systems. A further finding that detonations occurred in mixtures of shock-heated oxygen with lead tetramethyl and tetraethyl, both established as inhibitors of detonations in internal combustion engines [182], is a salutary reminder of the caution required in the choice of additives.

There has been little work on the effects of additives on the detonation of gases and vapours in the absence of oxygen. In the main the available information comes from experiments on mixtures of additives with acetylene, and this is confined to measurements of the minimum additions required to prevent the explosive decomposition of acetylene in small vessels [183]. As with the inhibition of confined detonations in oxyhydrogen mixtures by nitrogen, large amounts of additive are required. Typical results are shown in Table 4.7. The mole fraction of diluent required decreases with increasing initial pressure of the mixture and does not seem to vary significantly with the chemical composition of the diluent. It is probable that even higher degrees of dilution may be required to prevent the propagation of detonations along long pipelines.

Table 4.7 Dilution by various additives to prevent explosive decomposition of acetylene in small vessels [183].

Initial pressure of C_2H_2 + diluent (MN m^{-2})	%CO_2	%N_2	%He	%H_2	%C_4H_{10}	%C_3H_8
0.20	85	77	81	81	92	90
0.24	77	68	69	69	89	87
0.45	67	53	52	51	83	80
0.62	62	47	45	42	81	76
0.79	59	45	42	39	79	74

4.9 Detonations in suspensions of dusts and droplet mists in oxidizing atmospheres

An experimental observation is that, as the droplet size in a fog of hydrocarbon droplets is decreased to below a critical diameter of 10 μm, their ignition and subsequent burning exactly parallels that of a premixed gas flame [184]. With small droplets ignition energies are similar to those for premixed flames, and individual flames surrounding each droplet are replaced by global flame. Thus, it is not surprising that confined fogs of this kind are detonable, although the reaction zone can be some four to five times wider than that in a gaseous mixture. It is worth noting that no work on spherical detonations in such mists has been reported, although there is every reason to believe that they should support unconfined detonations. Again there is little or no data available on the detonation limits of confined clouds of this kind [185]. However, this may not be of great practical importance. The production of a monosize aerosol of droplets ≤10 μm in diameter requires extremely rigorous experimental procedures, so that they are unlikely to be encountered under normal conditions. For reasons discussed later in this section, it is not possible to predict confidently the contribution to a detonation made by the oversize fraction of droplets in the more probable wide size distribution of a fog generated in more usual conditions.

More recently it has become clear that confined fogs of droplets of hydrocarbons of diameter ≥1 mm in oxygen are readily detonable [186–195]. Nettleton [196] has reviewed this work and noted that there is general agreement that such detonation waves involve the break-up of the droplets. However, there is still some debate as to the importance of the various possible mechanisms involved in the shattering of the droplets. Presently little which is directly applicable to considerations of the safety of plant is known about the features of detonations in aerosols. Reaction zones, behind which expansion waves are generated, are generally wider and at a greater distance behind the leading shock, so that the duration of the peak pressures generated are up to ten times longer than those produced by gaseous mixtures. Detonation velocities can be as much as 50% below the Chapman–Jouguet value, calculated on the basis of the reaction of the complete charge of fuel. Thus, the internal pressures and their durations are generally below those produced by comparable gaseous mixtures. There have been no systematic studies of the composition limits for detonation in fogs with droplets of diameters ≫10 μm and little is known of the effects of replacing oxygen by air or of the use of an alternative gaseous oxidant.

It is becoming clear that the existence of the fuel phase in extremely fine form, involving the break-up of large aggregates of particles of the fuels or even individual particles, is not a prerequisite of the formation of a detonation. Thus, confined clouds of aluminium dust in oxygen [197], possibly also unconfined suspension in air [198, 199], confined suspensions of coal dust

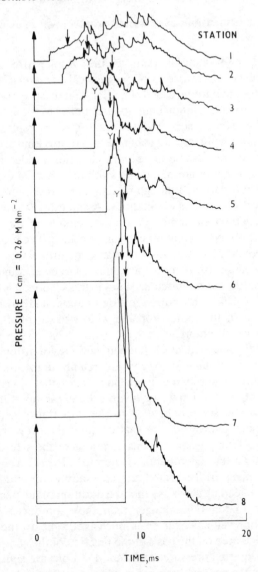

Figure 4.8 Development of pressure profiles in a coal dust–oxygen detonation, with ignition close to station 1; position of flame front marked by arrows [200].

in oxygen [38, 200], and probably clouds of corn dusts in both oxygen and air [201] will support detonation waves. Figure 4.8 illustrates the development of a detonation wave in a confined cloud of coal dust in oxygen [200]. It consists of a series of pressure histories taken at increasing distances from an igniter at the top of a vertical tube. As the leading front is amplified in its passage down the tube, the flame front, the position of which was determined by a series of photodiodes, gradually catches up with it to produce a fully-fledged detonation by station 7. By station 8, the detonation front, although still accelerating, approaches the expected C–J velocity.

The majority of the above studies have involved the use of particles of up to 100 μm in diameter, the rapid disintegration of which is difficult to conceive. Indeed, pronounced swelling of coal particles during their devolatilization is more probable at these high rates of heating [202]. However, there is some evidence to suggest that the transition to detonation occurs more readily with particles of diameters approaching 10 μm. Although most of the earlier experiments were carried out in oxygen atmospheres, more recent experiments have shown that detonations can be produced in suspensions of coal dusts in mixtures of oxygen and nitrogen at mole fractions of oxygen as low as 0.3 [203]. Indeed, measurements of the acceleration of flames in clouds of coal dust in air suggest they may be sufficient to produce a detonation in a long-enough tube [38]. There is also some evidence that additions of gaseous fuels in amounts which are well below the lower limit of flammability of the gas can transform non-detonable suspensions of dusts into detonable ones [204].

There have been few systematic studies of the composition and pressure limits for detonations in heterogeneous systems. One reason for this is the possibility of their becoming self-fuelling processes. Thus, it is known that wall films of hydrocarbons can be dispersed and ignited in the flow behind a shock [114], and in suitable circumstances fuel a gas-phase detonation [190]. The requisite conditions for the transformation of such a flame into a detonation have been analysed [205]. Again for dusts, experiments in mine galleries have shown that airstreams with velocities ≥ 30 m s^{-1} disperse deposits of coal dust from the walls and floor to produce a flammable suspension [115]. Thus, a combination of an igniter with a localized packet of flammable mixture which is sufficiently powerful to create a dispersion of fuel ahead of the initial flame can result in the production of a detonable medium, even in the absence of a primary suspension within the flammability limits. The difficulties in devising an experiment to measure the absolute composition limits for detonation in heterogeneous systems will readily be appreciated. In addition to the potential problems associated with the possibility of dispersion of fuels from the walls, further difficulties are produced by the continuous variation in the velocity of the leading front. Because of differences in the drag coefficients of the particles, they will accelerate at different rates, depending on their size and shape. Thus a single measurement of the density of the suspension prior to its ignition is not sufficient to define an absolute limit.

These cautionary remarks should be borne in mind when examining experimental measurements of limits [38], such as those shown in Fig. 4.9. This shows the velocities of a shock measured towards the end of a tube of limited length containing a suspension of coal dust in various mixtures of

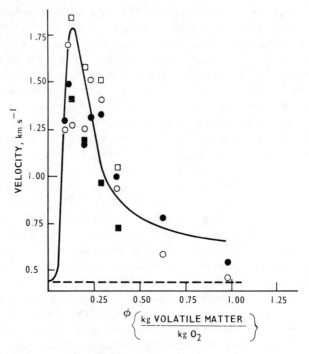

Figure 4.9 Influence of volatile content and particle size on velocity of detonations in coal dust–O_2–N_2 mixtures [38]. $\bigcirc,\bullet$ 54 μm dust, final and G2 velocities; $\square,\blacksquare$ 25 μm dust, final and G2 velocities; $---$ velocity in absence of coal dust.

oxygen and nitrogen. It was ignited by a detonation wave travelling from a stoichiometric mixture of acetylene and oxygen. The velocity of the resultant shock in the absence of a reaction between the coal dust and oxygen is shown by the horizontal line at about 0.4 km s^{-1}. Although the shock in reacting clouds is still accelerating towards the end of the tube (shown by the comparison of velocities at pressure measurement station G2 and the final measuring station), the plot of velocity versus the stoichiometry of the mixture, based on the mass of volatiles released from the initial composition of the cloud ϕ, serves to define a clear fuel-lean limit. The rate of change of velocity with stoichiometricity at low values of ϕ is similar for both sizes of particles. However, more experimental evidence is required before any firm conclusions can be drawn about the influence of the diameter of the particles on the composition limit.

As was the case with thermally-unstable fuels in the absence of oxygen (with the possible exceptions of unconfined clouds of aluminium dust in the presence of a powerful initiator [195, 196]), there are no well-authenticated recorded examples of unconfined detonations in heterogeneous systems.

However, there is some evidence for the possible occurrence of partly-confined detonations in aerosols of hydrocarbons [185, 193–195]. It is tempting to argue that the wider separation of precursor front and reaction zone in most heterogeneous systems compared with gaseous systems inhibits energy transfer. Allied to the requirement of creating fresh structure of an expanding front, such a constraint might well preclude spherical fronts in both heterogeneous mixtures and self-decomposing fuels. However, until a fuller understanding of the mechanisms is achieved, it would be inadvisable to base a safety case on such contentions. Further experimental studies on the possibility of expanding detonations in very fine mists which burn as premixed flames should produce some insight into the factors which apparently inhibit the initiation of spherical detonations in the case of heterogeneous mixtures and fuels in the absence of oxygen.

5

Initiation of a detonation wave

5.1 General remarks

Zel'dovich and Kompaneets strongly recommended that a standard procedure be adopted to study the formation of detonations in confined media [3]. They suggested the use of a long tube in which the mixture to be tested is separated from a readily-detonable mixture, with a well-defined detonation velocity, by a diaphragm. By removing the diaphragm some seconds before setting off a detonation in the driving mixture, diffusion across the interface ensures smooth propagation of the wave into the test medium. Variation of the composition and initial pressure of the driving mixture allows a check to be made on the influence of the strength of the triggering wave on the detonability of the medium to be tested. Happily, such techniques are being extended to unconfined detonations, using an abrupt expansion nozzle.

Unfortunately, a wide variety of sources with very different properties, the relationships between which are by no means clear, have been used in earlier studies of the formation of detonation waves. These have included charges of various condensed explosives, focused laser beams, electrically exploded wires and foils and conventional electrical discharges. The prospects of clarifying the relationships between energy deposited by such sources and identifying the mechanisms through which they originate detonations are not promising. Thus, an answer to the key question of the minimum energy requirements for a given source to trigger a detonation in a medium of prescribed temperature, pressure and composition is not likely to emerge for some time. Other factors contribute to this unsatisfactory situation: for instance, there is some suggestion that the transition to detonation is a stochastic process [206, 207]. Again, most experimental studies have involved the use of readily-detonable fuels, or of mixtures well away from the pressure and composition limits of detonability. It has by no means been established that the mechanisms governing the formation of a detonation in readily detonable media are relevant to initiation in marginally-detonable media.

Frequently the scale of the experiments has been such that it has been impossible to rule out the possibility of lasting effects from an energetic source or from the reflection of precursor blast waves from the confinement.

In the absence of a systematic approach to the problem, we have chosen an arbitrary division between strong and weak sources. This is convenient in that strong sources, namely those which produce a shock or blast wave of greater velocity than the C–J velocity of the test medium, are generally associated with unconfined media and with marginally-detonable systems. Consequently, the properties of different types of strong source are reviewed and compared with one another, to set in proper context available data on the critical energies required to initiate directly a spherical detonation. Incidentally, these energies can range from ≤10 J for sparks and exploding wires to ≤50 kJ for charges of condensed explosives. The demarcation allows for the natural introduction of information on minimum ignition energies (Section 5.5) and laminar burning velocities (Section 5.6) relevant to initiation by weak sources. It should be noted that, in contrast with critical energies required to produce a detonation, minimum ignition energies are typically tens of millijoules. Properties relating to flammability (Sections 5.5 to 5.7) are allied to those concerning detonability in a section dealing with the formation of shock and detonation waves by accelerating flames (Section 5.8). This concept is shown to be capable of producing some guidance on the distance required for a detonation to form in a number of confined mixtures of fuel and oxygen. Furthermore, the analysis, which requires a knowledge of only the laminar burning velocity and expansion ratio (Section 5.7) of the mixture, predicts the expected rapid increase in formation distances with composition, as fuel-lean and fuel-rich limits are approached. Presently, because of lack of experimental data, this method has only been validated for mixtures confined in tubes of small diameter (≤25 mm).

The division into strong and weak initiation results in some difficulties in choosing the appropriate section for certain aspects of initiation. For instance, there have been a number of suggestions as to the mechanisms whereby a flame in a large unconfined cloud of vapour might accelerate to produce a detonation, along with a number of experimental results on the critical mass of condensed explosive necessary to produce a spherical detonation. Thus detonation in unconfined clouds of vapour is treated separately in Section 5.4. Finally, on account of the paucity of experimental evidence, we have chosen to neglect the possibility of photochemical initiation of a detonation, although it may be of some import in, for example, mixtures of hydrogen and halogens.

5.2 Initiation of confined detonations by shock waves

Although the initiation of detonations by sparks and charges of condensed explosives also involves ignition in a shocked flow, we have chosen to deal with the subject separately. A brief explanation of the reasons for this may be helpful. Essentially the well defined and steady flow field behind a planar shock, propagating at a uniform velocity, results in major simplifications in the analysis of ignition and the subsequent transition to detonation. Experimental studies of this kind have done much to improve our understanding of the mechanisms governing the formation of a detonation wave. This contrasts with the much more complex situation presented by the time- and position-dependent flow field produced by blast waves from sparks and charges of condensed explosives. During the ignition phase, successive shells of the combustible mixture at increasing distance from the point at which the energy has been deposited are compressed and heated to progressively lower densities and temperatures.

The creation of detonations in confined media, behind both incident and reflected shock waves, has been widely studied [208–218]. From a practical viewpoint, the ideal result of such work would be the identification of a relationship between the ignition delay and the density and temperature, expressed in Arrhenius terms of the media behind a shock front travelling at the C–J velocity. Thus, the jump in temperature and pressure in the shocked gas defined by the C–J velocity, could be used in conjunction with experimental results on the influence of these parameters on ignition delays as a definition of detonability. However, experimental studies of shock initiation have clearly identified two forms of ignition which can occur in the heated and compressed medium. With initiating shocks of velocity well below that of a C–J wave, ignition generally occurs as a number of hot spots distributed randomly through the medium [219]. This has resulted in grave difficulties in producing an analysis of the formation of a detonation wave from a weakish source [220]. Such a treatment must incorporate a description of the manner in which the blast waves from individual pockets coalesce to form a second shock which, on merging with the original shock, should eventually result in a detonation. A further problem, common to ignition by both weak and strong shocks, concerns our lack of knowledge about the mechanisms which result in the eventual formation of the complex structure of transverse waves on an established detonation front. For instance, experimental studies have shown that a leading shock in mixtures of hydrogen and oxygen, diluted by argon, can be enhanced to velocities considerably in excess of C–J, without the development of the characteristic structure of a detonation front [221].

Despite the difficulties involved in producing a quantitative description of the origin of a detonation in a shocked gas, the experimental work of Oppenheim and co-workers [87, 90, 222] on shocks in explosive mixtures of gases has resulted in a clear insight into the various mechanisms which can trigger the transition from deflagration to detonation. These involve an 'explosion within an explosion' developing in the highly turbulent region between the leading shock front and the flame, with the resultant compression

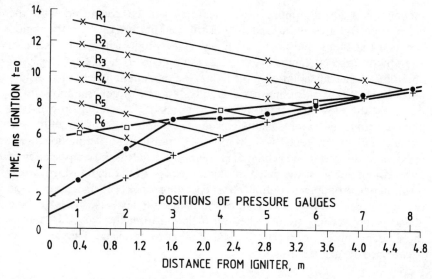

Figure 5.1 x–t diagram illustrating an 'explosion within an explosion' as a second flame ignites between stations 3 and 4 in a suspension of coal dust in oxygen [200]. + leading shock; ● flame front; □ pressure wave 'Y'; × reflected pressure waves 'R'.

fronts overtaking and merging with the precursor front, to form the detonation wave [223]. A similar mechanism operates in the formation of detonations in suspensions of coal dust in oxygen [200]. Figure 5.1 is a distance–time plot of the various peaks produced on recordings of pressure and light-emission from a number of measuring stations along the length of a vertical tube which contains a suspension of coal dust in oxygen. Clearly an 'explosion within an explosion' develops between stations 3 and 4 where there is an abrupt acceleration of the flame to a value approaching that of the leading shock front. However, other mechanisms can also operate in suspensions of dust. These seem to be related with the burning of the cloud in two stages. The initial flame consumes the readily volatilized portion of the particles, and the second results from the surface burning of the residues [224–226]. Whilst 'explosions within explosions' are likely to be the most common triggering mechanisms, the interaction of the precursor shock with a pocket of flame in the medium ahead of it can also transform a deflagration into a detonation.

Secondary explosions have been found to originate at the flame front itself, close behind the leading shock and at contact surfaces that are produced by collisions with secondary shocks. On occasion a volumetric explosion of the compressed flow may occur. It is reasonable to assume that the origin of the secondary explosion is governed by the shape and orientation of the leading shock and by the development of shocks moving transversely through the shocked flow. Furthermore, these features will be connected with the occurrence and growth of randomly distributed perturbations in the region between the shock and flame. Although some progress has been made in attempts to predict changes in shape of the precursor shock [227], brought about by surface instabilities in the flame, the random nature of such instabilities suggest that such analyses are unlikely to be of general application. Arguably the most important findings in terms of detonations in chemical plant are that any features likely to promote the formation of instabilities in either the flame or shock will promote the transition to detonation. Such features could include: (1) changes in composition across the cross-section of the medium ahead of the flame or along the path of the flame which would result in perturbations to both flame and leading shock; (2) changes in shape or size of the confinement ahead of the flame; (3) pockets of the medium ahead of the leading front ignited by radiation from the flame. However, there seems little prospect of designing plant to eradicate completely the occurrence of such features.

5.3 Initiation by blast waves from electrical and laser sparks and from charges of conventional explosives

This area has generated a great deal of experimental work [228], partly on account of the apparent simplicity of the experimental techniques and partly because of an implicit assumption that such sources resemble those to be found in plant. Furthermore, the attractive prospect of ranking detonability of various media and of different compositions of combustible mixture with a well-defined critical energy, produced by a spark, is evident. However, as will become apparent, these studies have not advanced our knowledge of critical energies required to produce detonations to a level comparable with that for minimum ignition energies of flammable mixtures. A number of factors contribute to this situation which deserve careful consideration, before the available data on critical energies for the production of a detonation are presented.

Experiments on spherical detonations have gone a considerable way towards identifying the important parameters controlling initiation by electrical sparks [122, 123, 229]. Thus, a widish gap, ~ 10 mm, was found to be required before the critical energy $E_c \sim 1$ J became independent of the shape of the electrodes and the width of the gap. This is explicable in terms of a relationship between the width of the gap and the spacing of transverse waves on the established front. Again, the critical triggering energy cannot be assigned a unique value, since it tends to a gradually decreasing level as the rate of energy deposition is increased; i.e. efficiency of transformation of electrical energy to kinetic energy of the surrounding medium increases as the rate of energy deposition increases to approach the ideal case of instantaneous deposition [230]. It is also worth noting that the critical energies were determined by integrating power–time curves for the discharges, apparently making no allowance for the efficiency of conversion of electrical energy into the production of blast waves. It has been shown that the efficiency in gaps of similar widths is less than 10% [231]. Nevertheless, such factors clearly indicate the dangers in regarding critical energies of electrical sparks as absolute quantities and the reservations necessary, when comparing different workers' results, involving different shapes of electrodes, different gap widths and various discharge circuits.

These reservations apply with even greater force to comparisons of initiation by electrical discharges with initiation by other strong sources. For instance electrically-fused wires [232, 233] and electrically-fused foils [234] have been used to generate detonations. Intuitively, the large expansion ratios associated with the vaporization of foils and wires should result in the production of stronger blast-waves. Certainly, experiments on the formation of spherical detonation waves using electrically-fused wires indicate that, by carefully optimizing conditions, up to 50% of the electrical energy could be converted to the formation of the initial blast-wave [232]. Again, features other than the influence of the strength versus distance characteristics of the initial blast-wave on the ignition of the surrounding medium could play an important role. For instance, variations in the emissivity of different types of source could well be important in igniting particles or droplets in two-phase systems. The nature and number density of active species, such as electrons with their high mobility, produced by different sources may also make a contribution to ignition. It is also conceivable that droplets and particles of metals and metallic oxides from exploding wires and foils could catalyse ignition. To date such features have not received due consideration.

There have been only a limited number of studies of laser-initiated detonations [128, 235–237]. At first sight this is somewhat surprising, in that the use of a laser obviates the potential influence of the surfaces of electrodes and of materials ejected from their surface on the generation of a detonation. Apparently these obvious advantages are outweighed by the experimental difficulties associated with requirement for accurate control of variations in the amount of energy dissipated.

Much of the experimental work on the composition limits of detonable unconfined clouds of vapour has been carried out using charges of conventional explosives. This is not to suggest that there is a suspicion that accidental explosions of this type have originated from such sources [1, 238], rather it has proved a convenient method of providing the required strengths of initiation to cover the range from readily-detonable to marginally-detonable mixtures. Although Tetryl has frequently been chosen as the condensed explosive, others have occasionally been employed. Table 5.1, from Kirk-Othmer [239], lists the relative efficiencies of a number of condensed explosives, both from the point of view of peak pressures and of durations of the positive impulse at a fixed distance from the charge. The latter parameter may have an important

Table 5.1   TNT equivalency (from Kirk-Othmer [239]).

Explosive	Pressure (%)	Impulse (%)
Lead ozide	30	35
Lead styphnate	80	65
Tetrazene	25	30
Nitroglycerine	135	120
Guanidine nitrate	100	65
Nitroguanidine	105	85
RDX slurry	155	155
Composition B	125	110
Composition A5	120	140
Black powder	50	50
Tetryl	120	130

bearing on triggering detonations in mixtures which are close to the limits, and consequently have longish induction distances between the leading front and reaction zone. Baker [240] gives similar information for an extended range of commercially-available explosives. At first sight differences of up to 50% in the relative efficiencies of the different explosives appear to be of similar significance to those for conversion of electrical energy to blast. However, the required mass of explosive may vary from ≤ 10 g for a readily detonable fuel in a stoichiometric mixture with oxygen to ~ 10 kg for a fuel such as methane in a stoichiometric mixture with air. Thus, corrections for the type of explosive are only likely to be of import in comparisons of readily-detonable mixtures. For example, Fig. 5.2 illustrates how the mass of explosive required varies with the composition of mixtures of ethylene and air [241]. Note that the energy released by Tetryl is $4.6 \, \text{kJ g}^{-1}$. Thus, even making appropriate allowances for the differences between mixtures with oxygen and air, there appears to be a considerable difference between the total energy required for initiation by electrical sparks and fuse wires and that required from charges of condensed explosives.

There have been few systematic studies of the effects of the nature of the triggering source. Charges of trinitrotoluene of mass $0.001 < m < 1$ kg have been used to produce spherical detonations in gaseous mixtures of fuel and air, and compared with an expanding spherical detonation wave used to set off spherical detonations in gaseous mixtures of fuel and oxygen [121]. For more readily-detonable fuels such as propane, the measured critical energy for initiation by an electrically-fused wire was $0.01 < E_c < 0.1$ J. However, the transition to detonation did not occur within the confines of the equipment either for less detonable fuels (e.g. methane) in mixtures with oxygen or for all fuels in mixtures with air. Since the main objective of this work [121] was to characterize the amplitude of the blast-wave produced in the surrounding

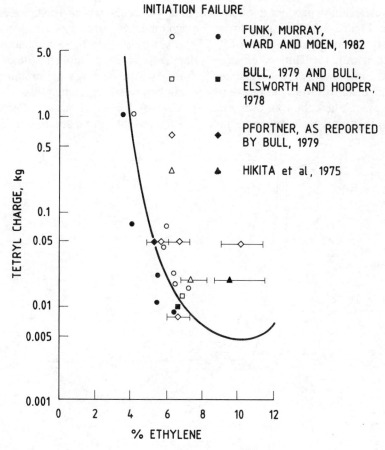

INITIATION FAILURE

○ ● FUNK, MURRAY, WARD AND MOEN, 1982

□ ■ BULL, 1979 AND BULL, ELSWORTH AND HOOPER, 1978

◇ ◆ PFORTNER, AS REPORTED BY BULL, 1979

△ ▲ HIKITA et al, 1975

Figure 5.2 Experimental determination of the fuel-lean limit of unconfined detonations of mixtures of ethylene and air (after Funk *et al.* [241]).

atmosphere, the comparison of the different sources was not extended further.

In order to take the question of a possible variation in energy of the source further, it is necessary to consider the mechanism through which a detonation is originated. It now appears to be generally accepted that the initiation of a spherical detonation from a source of lowish energy (e.g. masses of condensed explosive ≤10 g or electrical sparks) involves the decay of the initial blast wave to a velocity below the C–J value for the mixture, before the onset of chemical reactions in the flow [242, 243]. There may well be a period during which the wave propagates at a quasi-steady velocity, before accelerating to approach the C–J value [244, 245]. Typically, the decay of the triggering blast-wave from a small charge of condensed explosive, and the subsequent acceleration to produce a spherical detonation, occurs within a distance of 10 cm. Figure 5.3 illustrates this for stoichiometric mixtures of oxygen and acetylene at initial pressures of 50, 25 and 15 torr initiated by 45 mg charges of lead azide [245]. Thus, when we consider media which are difficult to detonate and consequently involve charges of >1 kg, we are dealing with initiation at large distances from the source (the strength of freely-expanding blast-waves decays as the cube root of the mass of charge). The large masses of charge together with the increased distances for the formation of a detonation leads

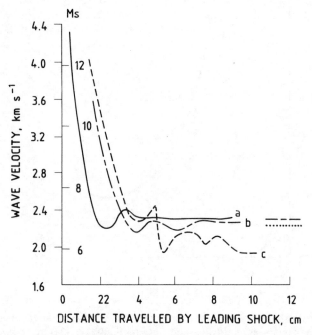

Figure 5.3 Microwave interferometric measurements of velocity of leading shock during the initiation of a spherical detonation in stoichiometric mixtures of oxygen with acetylene by a 75 J explosive charge (after Edwards *et al.* [245]). (a) $p_0 = 50$ torr; (b) $p_0 = 25$ torr; (c) $p_0 = 15$ torr; C–J velocities, ———$p_0 = 50$ torr, $\cdots\cdots p_0 = 10$ torr.

to the possibility of directional effects in the blast, caused by inhomogeneities in the charge and reflections of the front, and could well result in non-spherical initiation with charges of high mass. Much further experimental work is required before the results for readily-detonable and marginally-detonable media can be securely combined in a single model of the mechanism of initiation.

Similar difficulties arise in attempts to relate results obtained using electrical sources with those from charges of condensed explosives. For instance, it has been suggested that a parabolic shock front is created by the energy released from hot electrons in the leader front, bridging gaps of ≥ 10 mm between the electrodes [246, 247]. It is conceivable that a detonation might be created by this shock or its reflection from the electrode, rather than by the wave which initially expands away in cylindrical symmetry from the hot channel. Again, measurements on blast-waves from spark channels suggest the wave first forms much closer to the path of the deposited energy, than does blast from a condensed explosive [231]. This may well be due to the absence of any phase change in the spark channel, resulting in much smaller factors of expansion.

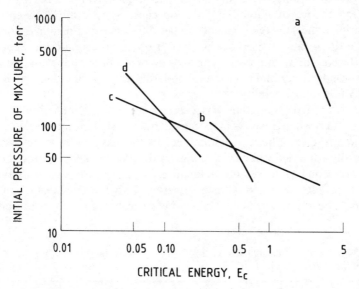

Figure 5.4 Influence of initial pressure and mode of initiation on critical energy, (a) $2H_2 + O_2$, electric spark; (b) $2C_2H_2 + 5O_2$ laser spark; (c) $2C_2H_2 + 5O_2$, expanding planar detonation; (d) $2C_2H_2 + 5O_2$, electric spark; a, b, d, E_c in J cm^{-1}; c, E_c in J. (After Sichel [249].)

Attempts to compare the probable efficiencies of spark channels and electrically-fused wires or foils reveal that the effects of a wide range of features are by no means understood. For instance, it is known that particles with appropriate drag coefficients and set into motion by a strong spherical blast-wave can overtake the more rapidly attenuating blast [248]. Thus, the possibility of ignition ahead of the original blast must be taken into account when considering exploding wires and foils. The effects of the production, on ignition, of highly mobile and possibly excited species such as electrons cannot be dismissed – Fig. 5.4 illustrates that (not unexpectedly) the critical energy of initiation differs markedly even for lasers and electric sparks [249]. It seems reasonable to expect even wider variations for fused wires and foils.

However, the marked increase in critical energy with decreasing initial pressure of the mixture should be noted.

There have been a number of semi-empirical treatments of the relationship between critical energies and the detonability of a medium. One such suggests that the critical energy for initiation by electrical and laser sparks and planar detonation waves decreases with decreasing initial pressure of gaseous mixtures [249]. A similar type of analysis has been applied to the prediction of composition limits for unconfined gaseous mixtures detonated by charges of condensed explosives; however, on account of the difficulties in relating the properties of various sources of initiation, it has proved impossible to produce a unified theory of initiation. Extreme caution therefore is essential in comparing critical energies obtained under different experimental conditions. Despite these cautionary remarks a set of observations on critical energies for different fuels, different compositions or different initial pressures of fixed composition, obtained from a standard source of initiation, can form a useful guide to detonability.

One set of such experiments has given a guide to the detonability of a wide range of fuels when mixed with oxygen [166]. The standard triggering source used to produce spherical detonations in the gaseous mixtures was an electrically-exploded wire. Table 5.2 gives the electrical energy stored in the capacitor required to set off detonations in the most readily detonable mixture of each fuel and oxygen, together with the composition of that mixture. The efficiency of conversion of electrical energy was measured and

Table 5.2 Critical initiation energies for spherical detonations in a variety of fuels mixed with oxygen [166].

Fuel	% (vol.) Fuel in most readily-detonable mixture	E_c (J)
Acetylene	40	<0.11
Ethyl nitrite	31	0.31
Propadiene	28.6	0.31
Methylacetylene	28.6	0.31
Ethylene oxide	40	0.31
Methyl vinyl ether	28.6	0.62
Cyclopropane	25	0.62
Ethylene	33	0.62
Vinyl fluoride	40	0.88
Propylene	25	1.25
Diethyl ether	20	2.5
Propane	22.2	2.5
Ethane	28.6	8.75
Acetaldehyde	40	12.5

found to be about 50%, so that the values of E_c are approximately half those tabulated [232].

There are two features of note in the data of Table 5.2. The mixture requiring the least energy to detonate is fuel-rich with respect to stoichiometry to steam and carbon dioxide as products of the reaction. Since increasing the percentage of fuel in the mixture will result in a lower specific heat ratio, the temperature and density behind a blast-wave from a given energy of source will be lower for fuel-rich mixtures. Thus, the lowered energies in fuel-rich mixtures must be due to the influence of composition on the chemistry of the initiating processes, rather than the properties of the initiating shock. As most work on initiation has been performed using stoichiometric mixtures, it is important to bear in mind that they are not necessarily the most easily detonable. The second feature concerns the wide variation in critical energy (two orders of magnitude) between acetylene and acetaldehyde, again indicating the importance of the chemical reactions, involved in initiation, in determining critical energies. Supporting evidence comes from work on the energy of explosive charge needed to trigger unconfined detonations in mixtures of propane, of butane, of propylene and of MAPP with air close to the fuel-rich limit [237]. Under these conditions the critical energy is related to the type of carbon–carbon bond in the fuel molecule. The anomaly between these results and the homology theory of limits for confined mixtures of fuel and oxygen is unresolved. It will be recalled that the homology theory involves the occurrence of extremely fast (and consequently non-rate-controlling) reactions, resulting in the formation of common fragments from a homologous series of parent fuel molecules. It seems highly improbable that the presence or absence of confinement is a significant factor, and the anomaly suggests that it would be unwise to extrapolate results from the homology theory from alkanes and alkenes of high molecular weight in mixtures with oxygen to other hydrocarbons in similar mixtures or to all hydrocarbons when mixed with air.

At the risk of some degree of trivialization it seems worthwhile summarizing the well-established features of strong initiation, which may be of some assistance in the safe design of chemical plant. At the outset it should be emphasized that the majority of the available information comes from experiments on gaseous mixtures of fuel and oxygen at equivalence ratios close to unity. In the absence of a unified theory, caution is evidently required when applying extrapolations of such data to fuel-lean mixtures with air, to two-phase systems and to self-decomposing media capable of supporting a detonation. It is evident that the chemical nature of the fuel strongly influences detonability. However, it is a gross oversimplification to think of this solely in terms of bond strengths in the fuel, both the carbon–carbon and carbon–hydrogen bonds in acetylene are considerably stronger than those in ethane, and yet critical energies for mixtures of acetylene and oxidant are approximately an order of magnitude less than for mixtures of ethane and oxygen. A general ranking order of hydrocarbons for ease of detonability would be the alkyne series, followed by (or possibly merging with) members of higher molecular weight of the alkene series. Cycloalkanes are probably more resistant to detonation than straight-chain alkanes and the gaseous alkanes of higher molecular weight are more prone to detonation in the presence of an oxidant than the lighter members of the series, with methane being highly-resistant to detonation. The fact that a fuel-rich limit appears to exist for mixtures of acetylene and oxygen suggests that spherical detonations may not occur in self-decomposing media. The possibility of spherical detonations in two-phase systems may well depend more on properties such as drag coefficient and particle size distribution, rather than on the chemical properties of particles and on those of any gases liberated from them. This is because the acceleration of the particles in the flow behind the initiating blast and consequently concentrations, etc. will depend on the former properties. Finally, it appears that, in terms of minimum requirements of energy, electrically-exploded wires or foils are potentially the most dangerous of possible initiating sources.

5.4 Detonation waves in large unconfined clouds of vapour

There has been only one reasonably well-authenticated example of a detonation in an unconfined cloud of vapour forming in air. This followed the ignition of a propane escape from a pipeline situated in a valley, so that the possibility of some effects arising from partial confinement cannot be completely excluded [250]. For other examples of explosions of unconfined clouds in which patterns of damage indicate the possibility of pockets of detonation, the confining effects of structures and buildings appear to have been of much greater import [251]. None the less, the possibility of the detonation of a truly unconfined cloud of vapour (as for example was considered in connection with the explosion at the Flixborough site in the UK in 1974) has excited great interest. Much interest has centred on the mechanisms whereby spherical flames can accelerate up to velocities of ≤ 100 m s^{-1} which are the minima necessary to account for the blast damage produced by the deflagration of a large cloud [252]. Recently, a number of hypotheses have been advanced, to account for either the possibility of a detonation [17] or for the acceleration of flames in large clouds [253–257]. Although the later hypotheses apply to deflagrations in the combustible mixture propagating at velocities approaching the speed of sound, continued acceleration of the flame through such mechanisms would lead to an eventual detonation.

The ingenious shock-wave amplified coherent energy release (SWACER) theory has recently been proposed to account for the direct formation of a spherical detonation [17]. However, there seems no reason why the model should not also apply to confined detonations. It involves the energy released from the igniting source producing an appropriate gradient of active species (such as free radicals or vibrationally-excited molecules) and of temperature, ahead of the advancing flame. Each successive shell of mixture treated by the spherically-expanding wave from a point source then has a different induction period, prior to the onset of exothermic reaction. It can readily be shown theoretically that, when the gradient of these induction periods is suitably related to the gradient of decay in velocity of the blast, the release of chemical energy couples to the leading front. This results in a rapid amplification of the front to the C–J value.

The potential rewards from the successful development of the theory, together with experimental confirmation that it is applicable to all forms of strong initiation, are evidently very high. Whilst it is possible to give an approximate estimate of the way in which a blast-wave from a variety of strong sources decays with distance from the origin, the difficulties in utilizing SWACER theory arise in defining the likely gradients in induction periods for the medium of interest. For the foreseeable future such information is only likely to be available for reactions in which the scheme of kinetics is simple and for which the gradient in temperature, rather than a gradient in concentration of active species, controls energy release. The use of the traditional technique of assessing hazard from readily-available information pertaining to weak initiation such as minimum ignition energies and flammability limits is thus likely to be necessary for some time to come.

Two further hypotheses have been advanced in order to account for the acceleration of flames in large clouds to approach sonic velocities. The two are not mutually exclusive and could well occur in combination in an explosion of a vapour cloud in the vicinity of a chemical plant. The first is concerned with the possible effects of intense radiation produced by large flames in pre-mixed clouds of gases [253–255]. The emissivity of such flames will be high on account of their optical depth. Presumably, similar effects should occur with smaller flames in suspensions of dusts and droplets on account of the higher emissivity of the particulate matter. Small-scale tests, with intensities of radiation about half that to be expected from a large cloud, have shown that incombustible fibrous particles can be sufficiently heated to serve as ignition centres ahead of the main flame front. With a probable random distribution of such particles in the atmosphere and on the ground surrounding a chemical plant, it can readily be appreciated that a succession of growing flamelets will result in greatly enhanced rates of flame propagation. An additional feature, which has not been considered, concerns the production of compression waves from individual flamelets. With a sufficient number of ignition centres, it is possible to visualize the production of a blast-wave, propagating on the gas ahead of the main flame, from the coalescence of such compression fronts. Certainly, the radiation hypothesis highlights the importance of careful housekeeping around chemical plant, in order to minimize the amount of fibrous material in its vicinity.

The second mechanism suggested to account for acceleration of flames in large clouds of vapour involves differences in the acceleration of pockets of burnt gases and pockets of the reactants in a turbulent flame [256, 257]. The differences arise from the effects of the mean gradients in pressure within the flame, principally due to buoyancy effects, acting on pockets of gas of different density. Further turbulence results, and a positive feedback mechanism is generated. The implications of this hypothesis to clouds with inhomogeneities in composition, to clouds with suspensions of the fuel in the form of droplets or particles and to clouds of self-decomposing fuels have not been explored. However, since the positive feedback mechanism depends on differences in density, the presence of inhomogeneities in the cloud could well enhance the acceleration of the flame. The practical implication is clear; any measures for alleviation of possible blasts should be designed to take effect before a turbulent flame can develop, preferably immediately following ignition of the cloud.

Methods of specifying parameters of a cloud, such as the composition, size and the scales and intensities of turbulence, necessary for the detonation of a large cloud, would obviously be of great value to designers of plant. Before parameters can be specified in a definitive fashion much work is required both in assessing the relative importance of the proposed mechanisms for acceleration of the flame and in obtaining further experimental data on the important parameters. Consider, for instance, the problem of defining the minimum diameter of a cloud for it to detonate (d_{min}). Experience of deflagrations in large clouds of vapour suggests that $d_{min} \geq 50$ m. An estimate of d_{min} can be approached via the radiation mechanism, by specifying the emissivity required to ignite pockets of the mixture ahead of the flame in predetermined times. However, appropriate data on ignition delays is required before the diameter of the initial flame can be calculated. Further information on, or assumptions about, the distribution of ignition sources ahead of this flame is necessary to account for the length scale associated with acceleration of the resultant flame. At present all that can be done is to make informed guesses about such data.

The following technique has been suggested for estimating d_{min} for mixtures for which either the spacing of transverse waves (S) on a steady-detonation or the relationship between induction time for the onset of exothermic reactions (τ) and temperature (T) is known [133]. It makes use of the experimental observation that the critical diameter (d_c) for reinitiation of detonations in stoichiometric mixtures of oxygen and acetylene in a tube with a sudden expansion in area is given by [32]

$$d_c = 13S \tag{5.1}$$

The experimentally determined relationship between the pitch of a spinning detonation (p) and the diameter of the containing tube [73]

$$p/d = 3 \tag{5.2}$$

suggests that, since spinning waves are generally associated with systems of marginal detonability,

$$d_{min} \geq 13S \geq 39d_c \tag{5.3}$$

For mixtures for which the relationship between induction period and gas temperature is known, d_{min} can be derived as follows. The induction periods for oxidation of gaseous mixtures of hydrocarbon and oxygen typically follow a law of the type

$$\log \tau [O_2]^n = A + (B/T) \tag{5.4}$$

where A and B are constants. This has been used to estimate the length of the induction zone (L_i) from

$$L_i = \tau M a_o \tag{5.5}$$

where M is the Mach number of the precursor shock (i.e. the C–J velocity) and a_o is the speed of sound in the mixture. Since for many gaseous mixtures

$$S \simeq 0.6 n L_i, \text{ where } 10^2 < n < 10^3 \tag{5.6}$$

d_{min} can be obtained from Equation 5.3.

Some comments on the probable accuracy of the predictions are appropriate – for instance, not all gaseous mixtures of oxygen and hydrocarbon behave according to Equation 5.1. Fuels more resistant to detonation result in higher values of d_c with $d_c \sim 18S$ for mixtures of either methane or acetone with oxygen at sub-atmospheric pressures. However, the uncertainties associated with the spread in values of $10^2 < n < 10^3$ in Equation 5.6 may be of greater import. These values of n are based on experiments with homogeneous gaseous mixtures of oxygen and hydrocarbon. The limits in the value of n may well be much wider for different oxidants and heterogeneous media. Presently the wisest course is to regard assessments of d_{min} as a useful yardstick for comparative purposes. In this context data on critical diameters have been collected in Table 5.3 and converted to values of d_{min} [258]. The measured values of E_c for each mixture are included in the table. The fact that the ranking order of fuels mixed with oxygen is followed by their mixtures with air lends some confidence to the predictions of d_{min}; furthermore, the values for mixtures with air are consistent with the minimal available evidence. The differences in critical energies, revealed by a comparison of the results for mixtures of various fuels with oxygen in Tables 5.2 and 5.3, are typical of the variations reported by different workers.

5.5 Minimum ignition energies

Minimum ignition energies (E_{min}) form an appropriate introduction to weak initiation of detonation waves. Preceding sections have illustrated that there is experimental information available on the detonability of only a limited

Table 5.3 Minimum cloud diameters and critical energies for unconfined detonations in mixtures of various fuels with oxygen and air [258].

Fuel	Oxidant	d_{min} (m) [14]	d_{min} (m) [259]	E_c (J) [259]
40% C_2H_2		>0.10	>0.04	$3.8 \times 10^{-4} < E_c < 10^{-2}$
40% C_2H_4O			>0.11	1.2×10^{-2}
33.3% C_2H_4			>0.20	7.2×10^{-2}
33.3% C_3H_6	O_2		>0.27	0.2
22.2% C_3H_8			>0.39	0.6
66.7% C_2H_6			>0.51	1.1
66.7% H_2		>0.74	>0.78	1.6
40% CH_4		>1.25	>1.95	51
12.5% C_2H_2			>3.12	1.3×10^2
12.3% C_2H_4O			>11.7	7.6×10^3
9.5% C_2H_4			>31.2	1.2×10^5
6.6% C_3H_6			>58.5	7.6×10^5
5.7% C_3H_8	Air		>85.8	2.5×10^6
5.7% C_2H_6			>109.6	5.1×10^6
29.6% H_2			>109.6	4.2×10^6
12.3% CH_4			>398	2.3×10^8

number of fuels (mainly gaseous ones) and on an even more limited range of oxidants. Therefore, when assessing potential hazards, it is often necessary to take recourse to the wider selection of data on flammability. In this context minimum ignition energies can be regarded as equivalent to critical energies for the initiation of unconfined detonations, giving a useful guide to the ranking of potential hazard. Fortunately, a wider understanding of the empirical relationship between minimum ignition energies and the properties of the medium is beginning to emerge from the work of Ballal and Lefebvre [260–265], so that it is possible to calculate their approximate magnitude for two-phase systems on which few, if any, experimental measurements have been made.

Minimum ignition energies are generally derived from measurements of electrical energy dissipated in a spark gap. Because of differences in the physical processes involved in heat and mass transport in spark channels and flames, a brief description of the concept of a minimum ignition energy is appropriate. It involves the electrical energy released in the gap producing a similar temperature gradient to that in a steadily propagating flame within, or close to, the gap. This presents some practical problems in the choice of the gap width, shape of electrodes and rate and duration of release of energy. The optimum values of these parameters must be determined experimentally, for instance with narrow gaps incipient flames are quenched by the losses to the electrodes and the optimum width of gap (d_{opp}) is generally about twice the maximum quenching distance (d_q). Again, the rate at which electrical energy is released within the gap controls the amount dissipated in the surrounding atmosphere, and consequently lost to the ignition process, in the formation of a blast-wave. So, when the gap width differs widely from d_{opp} or rates of energy release are high enough to approximate to instantaneous release of energy, up to ten times E_{min} may be necessary for ignition. Nevertheless, experimental determinations or theoretical predictions of E_{min} are a useful guide to the relative hazards associated with fuels for which the detonable characteristics are unknown. In this context Ballal's treatment [265] is particularly useful, since it relates E_{min} with fairly readily-available information on the physical properties of the fuel. Figure 5.5 shows a compilation of minimum ignition energies for a variety of stagnant, two-phase and homogeneous mixtures of stoichiometric composition with air at atmospheric pressure. Droplet and particle sizes for the heterogeneous mixtures were about 50 μm. The results correlate well with the Spalding mass transfer number B:

$$B = \frac{q_{st}H + c_{pa}(T_g - T_b)}{L + c_p(T_b - T_s)} \tag{5.7}$$

where q_{st} = mass ratio of fuel to air in a stoichiometric mixture
$\quad\quad H$ = heat of combustion
$\quad c_{pa}$ = specific heat of air
$\quad\; c_p$ = specific heat of fuel
$\quad\quad L$ = latent heat of evaporation of fuel
$\quad\; T_g$ = gas temperature
$\quad\; T_b$ = boiling point of the fuel
$\quad\; T_s$ = surface temperature of the fuel.

An approximate estimate of E_{min} for stoichiometric mixtures can be obtained by calculating B from Equation 5.7 and reading the corresponding value for E_{min} from Fig. 5.5.

For a more accurate estimate of E_{min} and the way in which it varies with composition of the mixture and size of the particle/droplet in two-phase media, Ballal [265] recommends the use of the following equations, for the quenching distance d_q

$$d_q = \sqrt{(8\alpha)} \left\{ \left[\frac{C_3{}^3 \rho_p D_{32}^2}{8C_1 f^2(k/c_p)\phi \ln(1+B)} + \frac{12.5\alpha}{S_u{}^2} \right]^{-1} - \frac{9qC_1{}^2 \epsilon\sigma T_p{}^4}{c_p \rho_p C_3{}^3 f D_{32} \Delta T_{st}} \right\} \tag{5.8}$$

and for E_{min}

$$E_{min} = \pi c_p \rho_a \Delta T d_q{}^3 \tag{5.9}$$

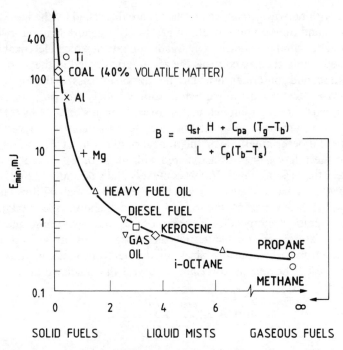

Figure 5.5 Theoretical minimum ignition energies for a range of fuels in air at $p_o = 1$ bar, $d = 50\ \mu$m, $\phi = 1$ and $T = 290$ K (after Ballal [265]).

where α = thermal diffusivity of fuel droplet/particle
     ρ = density
     ϵ = emissivity of particle/droplet
     ϕ = equivalence ratio
     σ = Stefan–Boltzmann constant
     C_1 = ratio of surface mean area to Sauter mean diameter
     C_3 = ratio of volume mean diameter to Sauter mean diameter
     c_p = specific heat of fuel
     D_{32} = Sauter mean diameter
     f = swelling factor of fuel
     k = thermal conductivity of fuel
     S_u = laminar burning velocity of the mixture
     T = temperature
    ΔT_{st} = temperature rise in a stoichiometric flame
subscripts a and p refer to air and fuel respectively.

The first term in brackets on the right hand side of Equation 5.8 represents diffusion, the second chemical reaction and the final term accounts for losses by radiation.

There have been numerous experimental studies of minimum ignition energies for stagnant mixtures of gases [8]. More recent measurements have resulted in somewhat lower values, as measurements of the power supplied to the arc have increased in accuracy [266, 267]. Arguably, the most comprehensive survey of methods of calculating minimum ignition energies comes from Ballal and Lefebvre [264] who give expressions for calculating the quenching distance for both homogeneous and heterogeneous mixtures in stagnant and flowing systems. Table 5.4 gives these expressions which can then be used with Equation 5.9 to calculate E_{min}.

It will be noted that values of burning velocity are required in order to derive E_{min}. The following section describes methods of predicting laminar burning velocities and S_t can be obtained from Equation 5.24. Possibly a more reliable relationship between S_t and S_u, which takes into account the existence of a plateau in S_t with increasing turbulence and which might be expected in view of eventual extinction at very high levels of turbulence is that suggested by Abdel-Gayed and Bradley [268] and shown as Fig. 5.7.

5.6 Laminar burning velocities

There is a relative wealth of information on the laminar burning velocities of gaseous fuels at atmospheric pressure and how these vary with the composition of the mixture, its oxygen content and nature of any diluent [8, 269]. However, similar information on heterogeneous and hybrid systems is scant. Recently Ballal [270] has suggested a method of calculating burning velocities of both homogeneous and heterogeneous systems. Figure 5.6 shows a very favourable comparison of his calculated values of burning velocity for a wide range of types of fuel with calculations based on the Spalding mass transfer number, B. There are good reasons for expecting a somewhat poorer performance of the theoretical treatment, when applied to less-idealized situations. For instance the experimental results are for monosize particles and droplets and gravitational effects were carefully excluded in the experiments. The range of laminar burning velocities of gaseous fuels is much wider in practice than the theoretical result of $40 < S_u < 45$ cm s^{-1}, indicated as B approaches infinity in Fig. 5.6.

Despite these cautions, Ballal's analysis [270] is of general applicability to a wide variety of practical situations, excluding those involving any contribution to heating of the mixture by radiation from hot surrounding walls. Thus, S_u is calculated from the thickness of the reaction zone (δ_r) given by

$$\delta_r = \alpha_g^{0.5} \left\{ \left[\frac{C_3^{3} \rho_f D_{32}^{2}}{8f^2 C_1 (c_p/k)_g \phi \ln(1+B)} + \frac{\alpha \Delta T_r}{S_g^{2} \Delta T_{pr}} \right]^{-1} - \frac{9qC_1^{2} \epsilon \sigma T_p^{4}}{c_{pg} \rho_f C_3^{3} f D_{32} \Delta T_r} \right\}^{-0.5} \tag{5.20}$$

Table 5.4 Equations for calculating quenching distances for various mixtures under different conditions [264].

Type of mixture	Equations	
Homogeneous, quiescent	$d_q = \dfrac{10\alpha}{S_u}$	(5.10)
Homogeneous, low turbulence	$d_q = \dfrac{10\alpha^{0.5}(\alpha + 0.08u'\,d_q)^{0.5}}{(S_u - 0.16u')}$	(5.11)
Homogeneous, high turbulence	$d_q = \dfrac{10\alpha}{(S_t - 0.63u')}$	(5.12)
Heterogeneous, monodisperse, quiescent, $t = 0$, $\Omega = 0$	$d_q = D_{32}\left[\dfrac{\rho_p}{\rho_a \phi \log(1+B)}\right]^{0.5}$	(5.13)
Heterogeneous, monodisperse, quiescent, t_c = finite	$d_q = \left[\dfrac{(1-\Omega)\rho_p D_{32}^2}{\rho_a \phi \log(1+B)} + \left(\dfrac{10\alpha}{S_u}\right)^2\right]^{0.5}$	(5.14)
Heterogeneous, polydisperse, quiescent, t_c = finite	$d_q = \left[\dfrac{C_3^{\,3}(1-\Omega)\rho_p D_{32}^2}{C_1\rho_a \phi \log(1+B)} + \left(\dfrac{10\alpha}{S_u}\right)^2\right]^{0.5}$	(5.15)
Heterogeneous, polydisperse, low turbulence, t_c = finite	$d_q = [1 + (0.08u'\,d_q/\alpha)]^{0.5}\left[\dfrac{C_3^{\,3}(1-\Omega)\rho_p D_{32}^2}{C_1\rho_a \phi \log(1+B)(1+0.25C_2^{0.5}\,Re_{\text{Dzz}}^{0.5})} + \left\{\dfrac{10\alpha}{(S_u - 0.16u')}\right\}^2\right]^{0.5}$	(5.16)

Heterogeneous, polydisperse, low turbulence, $t_c = 0$

$$d_q = [1 + (0.08u' d_q/\alpha)]^{0.5} \left[\frac{C_3^3(1-\Omega)\rho_p D_{32}^2}{C_1\rho_a\phi\log(1+B)(1+0.25C_2^{0.5}Re_{D_{32}}^{0.5})} \right]^{0.5}$$

(5.17)

Heterogeneous, polydisperse, high turbulence, $t_c =$ finite

$$d_q = \frac{0.32Pr(1-\Omega)\rho_p D_{32}^{1.5} u'^{0.5}}{Z\rho_a^{0.5} \mu_a^{0.5} \phi\log(1+B)} + \frac{10\alpha}{(S_t - 0.63u')}$$

(5.18)

Heterogeneous, polydisperse, high turbulence, $t_c = 0$

$$d_q = \frac{0.32Pr(1-\Omega)\rho_p D_{32}^{1.5} u'^{0.5}}{Z\rho_a^{0.5} \mu_a^{0.5} \phi\log(1+B)}$$

(5.19)

$\Omega =$ fraction of fuel in the form of vapour
$\nu =$ kinematic viscosity
$\mu =$ dynamic viscosity
$\mu_a =$ viscosity of air
$C_2 =$ ratio of mean diameter to Sauter mean diameter
$Pr =$ Prandtl number ($c_p\mu/k$)
$Re_{D_{32}} =$ $u' D_{32}/\nu$
$Z =$ $C_1 C_2^{0.5}/C_3^3$
$S_u =$ laminar burning velocity
$S_t =$ turbulent burning velocity
$u' =$ r.m.s. of fluctuating velocity
Other symbols are as defined previously.

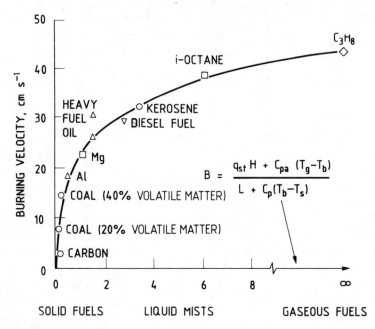

Figure 5.6 Laminar burning velocities of fuel–air mixtures for which physical processes dominate propagation $d = 30$ μm; $p_o = 1$ bar; $T = 290$ K; $\phi = 1$. (After Ballal [270].)

and for the laminar burning velocity from

$$S_u = \frac{\alpha \Delta T_r}{\delta_r \Delta T_{pr}} \qquad (5.21)$$

In equation 5.20, subscript g is used for gas and S_g is the laminar burning velocity of the gases liberated from the particles/droplets of fuel. In the case of metallic particles, such as aluminium and magnesium, which burn as metal vapours are released into the gas phase, S_g is the laminar burning velocity of the vapour phase flame. For materials such as coal, carbon, predominantly hydrocarbon-based plastics, flour dusts, etc., the rate of burning of which is essentially controlled by the slow oxidation of carbon monoxide in the gas phase, the use of the laminar burning velocity of carbon monoxide has been recommended. In evaluating equation 5.20, it is necessary to use values of (k, c_p and ρ)$_g$ at a temperature intermediate between that of the ignition and that of the reaction zone. The symbols of Equations 5.20 and 5.21 retain their previous significance and subscripts r and pr refer to reaction and pre-ignition zones respectively.

Finally, a brief guide to the likely magnitudes of laminar burning velocities

Table 5.5 Typical values of laminar burning velocities.

Fuel/mixture	S_u in absence of oxidant $(m\,s^{-1})$	S_u in air $(m\,s^{-1})$	S_u in oxygen $(m\,s^{-1})$
Self-decomposing fuels e.g. C_2H_2	>0.1		
Particulate suspensions		$0.05 < S_u < 0.2$	Slight increase since the effect of the higher temperature of the flame is compensated by much higher radiation losses
Droplet fogs		$0.2\ < S_u < 0.35$	Increase by a factor of ≤ 2, since radiation losses are limited by the lowish boiling points of most fuels
Hybrid fog and vapour		$0.3\ < S_u < 0.4$	Similar increase by a factor of ~2
Homogeneous gaseous mixtures		<0.5*	$1.0 < S_u < 4.0$†

*Stoichiometric mixtures of hydrogen and air and acetylene and air $S_u > 1.0\,\mathrm{m\,s^{-1}}$
†Stoichiometric mixtures of hydrogen and oxygen and acetylene and oxygen $S_u \sim$ $10\,\mathrm{m\,s^{-1}}$

to be anticipated in different systems is given in Table 5.5. The results for all but the homogeneous mixtures of gases came from Ballal [270]; for the latter mixtures experimental results are given. The influence of the initial pressure and temperature of the medium on predicted burning velocities depends on the relative importance of the mass transfer term (the first term in square brackets in Equation 5.20), the chemical term (the second in square brackets in 5.20) and the term describing radiation losses. A survey of experimental measurements of S_u of mixtures of methane and air [271] has assumed that S_u varies as the square of the initial temperature of the mixture. There is no experimental evidence on the influence of initial pressure and temperature on the laminar burning velocity of heterogeneous mixtures.

5.7 Expansion ratios

At this stage it is convenient to deal with expansion ratios, ϵ, the ratio of the density of the unburnt mixture to that of the products. They are used later in the text in terms of the early stages of acceleration of flames. Obviously ϵ depends on the flame temperature (T_f) and any change in the number of moles of products relative to those of reactants; with heterogeneous systems there is a significant contribution from the change in phase of fuel; the final temperature of the flame is governed by the heat of combustion or of decomposition of the particular fuel and the composition of the mixture. However, it is possible to give some approximations which apply to a range of gaseous fuels and (less securely) to heterogeneous systems. For mixtures of fuel and air close to stoichiometric composition, flame temperatures are typically about 2300 K, and for similar mixtures with oxygen about 3300 K. For mixtures close to the fuel-lean limit of flammability flame temperatures lie in the range $1600 \text{ K} < T_f < 1900 \text{ K}$, with the lower end of the temperature range applicable to fuels of low molecular weight. Similar generalizations should apply to fogs of droplets sufficiently small in diameter ($\leq 10 \ \mu$m) to burn as premixed systems, and probably to suspensions of fine dusts which volatilize at temperatures well below that of the flame to produce a flammable vapour, for example coal dust [272, 273]. For metal dusts which volatilize at high temperatures and for largely non-volatile carbonaceous particles, losses by radiation will result in a decrease in flame temperatures.

In assessing potential hazards the most commonly encountered situation is a fuel-lean mixture with air. For homogeneous mixtures this effectively minimizes any change in the number of moles of products relative to those of reactants. However for self-decomposing fuels such as ozone and hydrogen peroxide and mixtures of high molecular weight hydrocarbons with oxygen, changes in the number of moles of products relative to those of the reactants can make an important contribution to the expansion ratio. With heterogeneous suspensions, the increase in volume due to gasification makes a more important contribution to the expansion ratio. Because it is impossible to specify the exact composition of gases liberated from materials such as coal, flour, hydrocarbon-based plastics (and indeed these may well vary with the rate of heating of the particles), it is impossible to generalize on the contribution gasification makes to the expansion ratio. Even for droplets of hydrocarbons, cracking of the parent fuel molecules in the gas phase may occur before their progeny burn and result in an increase in the expansion ratio. Each case *must* be considered on an individual basis.

5.8 Detonations arising from accelerating flames

Although experimental studies of detonation waves are generally carried out using strong initiation (mainly to reduce the size of the equipment), accidental detonations in and around chemical plant are frequently associated with initiation involving an accelerating flame. Consequently, theoretical treatments of the development of a detonation from an initial flame, and how this might vary with the properties of the medium and type of confinement, assume considerable import in practice. Of particular interest is the distance between the ignition of a flame and the formation of a steady detonation wave. For instance, it is possible to consider the design of a plant in which the lengths of runs of pipework are kept below the minimum formation distances for any compositions or pressures of the media likely to be encountered in practice. Again, the formation distance for a steady detonation indicates where flame inhibitors and arresters are likely to be effective and in conjunction with an estimate of the average velocity over the distance gives the time available for the dispersal of a flame suppressant. Finally, the possibility of pressure-piling, a process leading to the production of abnormally high pressures, increases with increasing run-up distances.

Run-up distances have been studied for a variety of gaseous fuels and a number of oxidants [172, 174, 177, 274, 275]. As the composition of the mixture approaches the limits of detonability, these distances might be expected to increase rapidly, offering a method of determining detonability limits. However, there have been few attempts to generalize from these studies in order to predict how parameters such as diameter of a pipeline should influence run-up distances [112, 276]. In this context, we have chosen to examine how an analysis of the formation of a shock-wave by a confined and accelerating flame might be extended to the production of a detonation. It will be shown to produce a useful guide both to the manner in which run-up varies with the nature of the fuel molecule and the composition of mixtures of fuel and oxygen.

The theory we use [112] treats the flame (of velocity v_f) as an accelerating piston which drives a velocity gradient in the unburnt medium from a gas velocity $U = \beta v_f$ immediately ahead of it, to a velocity $U = 0$ at the position which the most distant pressure wave has reached. The resultant equations can be solved by assuming various values of the constant β. The appropriate value will depend on the shape and structure of the flame, but $\beta = 0.9$ is a popular choice. Solutions for the time and distance at which a shock is first formed are available for flames with: (1) accelerations $g_f = dv_f/dt = $ constant [277]; (2) acceleration increasing with time squared, $g_f = k^2 t^2$, [277] where k is a constant and t time and (3) acceleration which increases exponentially with time, $g_f = v_{fo} e^{ct}$ [278] where v_{fo} is the initial velocity of the flame and c a constant. For present purposes the use of $g_f = $ constant suffices to estimate the distance from the origin of the flame to its position at the time at which the shock first forms (X_f), and from the origin to the position at which the shock is produced (X_s), in terms of the specific heat ratio of the reactants (γ), the speed of sound in the uncompressed reactants (c), the ratio of the velocity of the flow immediately ahead of the flame to that of the flame, β and the acceleration of the flame (g_f) as

$$X_f = \frac{2c^2}{(\gamma + 1)^2 \beta^2 g_f} \tag{5.22}$$

and

$$X_s = \beta(\gamma + 1)X_f \tag{5.23}$$

Thus a yardstick, involving readily-available data on the unburnt medium, exists for estimating the run-up distance for a detonation, X_d, provided that a relationship can be developed between X_s and X_d.

Such a relationship can probably be most readily appreciated from a description of the various processes which lead to the acceleration of flames in media confined in tubes with smooth walls. In the early stages of burning the velocity of the flame will increase because of the confinement of the products. In this initially spherical phase of propagation the velocity of the flame will be related to the product of the laminar burning velocity and the expansion ratio, $\epsilon (= \rho_u/\rho_b)$. Typically, for detonable media $\epsilon S_u \leq 15$ ms^{-1}. As the flame approaches the walls a flow of the reactants will develop, adding to the velocity of flame propagation. Further acceleration may also occur at this stage through an increase in area of the flame. As the flow of reactants accelerates, turbulence will develop, resulting in a further acceleration of the flame appropriate to the turbulent burning velocity, S_t.

Various relationships between S_u and S_t have been proposed. One which is commonly used is

$$S_t = S_u + \left\{ 2S_u u' \left[1 - \frac{S_u}{u'} (1 - e^{-u'/S_u}) \right] \right\}^{0.5} \tag{5.24}$$

where u' is the velocity scale of turbulence. Typically the ratio S_t/S_u can increase with increasing u' to $S_t/S_u \leq 15$. Note that Fig. 5.7, showing a

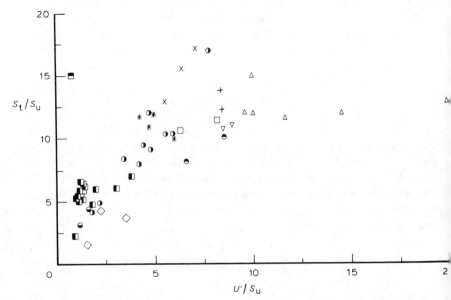

Figure 5.7 Experimental studies of relationship between turbulent and laminar burning velocities, $500 \leq \mathrm{Re} \leq 750$ (after Abdel-Gayed and Bradley [268]).

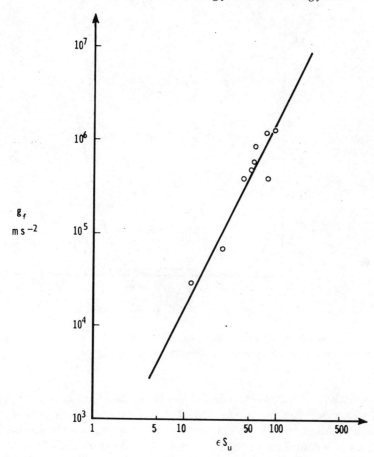

Figure 5.8 Induction times and distances for transition to detonation in confined mixtures, expressed as effective acceleration of the flame [279].

compilation of various experimentalists' results (denoted by the different symbols) of the effect of u' on S_t, [268] shows that further increases in u' are ineffective in raising the value of S_t. Such behaviour is implicit in the concept of extinction through excessive stretch of the flame at high levels of turbulence.

Analysis indicates that a shock first forms as the velocity of the flame approaches the speed of sound in the uncompressed reactants, say for fuel-lean mixtures $v_f \sim 300$ m s^{-1}. There are fairly wide variations in the laminar burning velocities of detonable media, say $0.5 < S_u < 5$ m s^{-1}, with the lower velocities corresponding to marginally-detonable mixtures and self-decomposing fuels. More readily-detonable mixtures should result in the formation of the shock prior to the achievement of the maximum value of

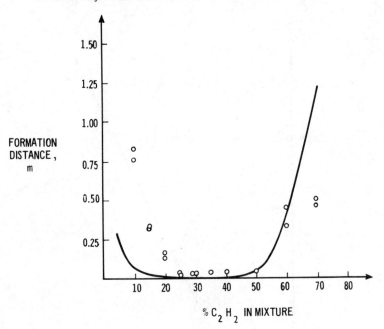

Figure 5.9 Comparison of measured run-up distances [177] in mixtures of acetylene and oxygen with predicted distances for shock formation [112].

flame velocity, so that acceleration of the flame continues during the transition phase between the production of the shock and the formation of a steady detonation. In addition, the heating of the compressed medium behind the shock will contribute to the acceleration of the flame. Such heating can result in a second flame igniting in the flow ahead of the original flame, possibly aided by the occurrence of pre-flame reactions conditioning the gas there [105]. With suspensions of dusts (and possibly droplets), the increased density will increase the effective absorption of radiation from the original flame and consequently the rate at which the particles approach their ignition temperature. It is therefore reasonable to assume that a major portion of the run-up distance for the formation of detonation waves is associated with the formation of the initial shock front.

The problem of predicting formation distances resolves itself into finding reliable estimates of the acceleration of flames and whether these vary with time. Pawel *et al.* [279] measured the times and distances required to produce detonations in a variety of fuels mixed with oxygen, air and nitrous oxide at a pressure of 1 bar in a narrow tube ($d = 26$ mm). Average values of acceleration derived from these are shown in a log–log plot of g_f versus ϵS_u in Fig. 5.8. Since S_u and S_t are related, for example through an equation of the type of Equation 5.24, the choice of S_u as the fundamental variable is not significant.

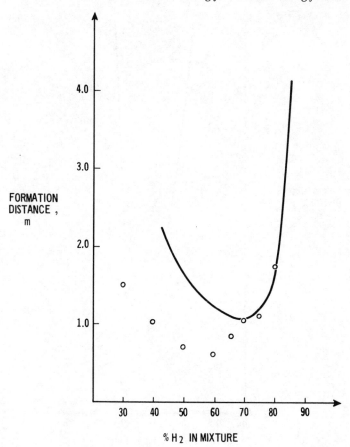

Figure 5.10   Comparison of measured run-up distances [177] in oxyhydrogen mixtures with predicted distances for shock formation [112].

Figure 5.8 shows an acceptably linear relationship between g_f and ϵS_u, allowing g_f to be derived for mixtures of fuel and oxidant confined in tubes of small diameter, when the appropriate laminar burning velocities and expansion ratios are known.

   In order to test the generality of the relationship between g_f and ϵS_u, we have compared predictions based on it with the experimental measurements of run-up distances for detonations and how these vary with the composition of the mixture obtained by a different set of investigators [177, 274]. In the main, these were obtained in a tube of smaller diameter (15 mm) than that on which Fig. 5.8 is based. Figures 5.9 to 5.11 show these comparisons of X_s, the lines on the plots, with X_d, the experimental points for mixtures of acetylene, hydrogen and methane respectively with oxygen. The values of X_s have been derived from Equations 5.22 and 5.28 with $\beta = 0.9$ and g_f from available data

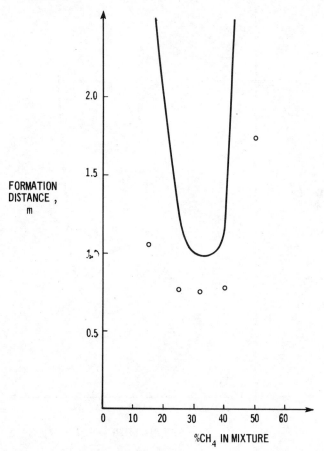

Figure 5.11   Comparison of measured run-up distances [177] in oxymethane mixtures with predicted distances for shock formation [112].

on S_u and ϵ. Not only do the curves representing X_s give tolerable estimates of X_d, but they also show the sharp increase in distance to be expected as fuel-lean and fuel-rich limits are approached. Indeed, they give a very good estimate of the fuel-rich limit; however, for oxyacetylene mixtures the predicted fuel-lean limit is too lean, and for methane and hydrogen it is on the side of fuel-richness. This could well be due to significant differences between the Lewis number (the ratio of thermal to mass diffusivity) appropriate to fuel-lean and to fuel-rich mixtures having significant effects on the acceleration of the flame. The limited comparison possible for mixtures of fuel and air and fuel with nitrous oxide at about 1 bar [172] suggests that tolerable but somewhat poorer estimates of X_d are obtained for detonations in tubes of small diameter. However, a combination of values of g_f from Fig. 5.8 with Equations 5.22 and 5.23 is unsatisfactory for gases which exothermically

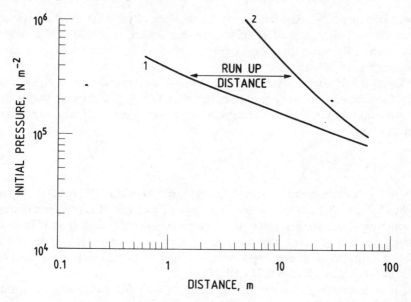

Figure 5.12 Effect of initial pressure on run-up distances for confined detonations in pure acetylene [174].

decompose in the absence of oxygen, predicting run-up distances up to ten times those observed experimentally. This is not unreasonable in that different mechanisms may well contribute to the acceleration of flames in self-decomposing media.

Acetylene is the only example of self-decomposing gases for which extensive data on run-up distances are available [174]. Figure 5.12 shows a compilation of the influence of the initial pressure on initiation distance. Line 1 represents the conditions resulting in the production of a deflagration and line 2 those for a detonation. The horizontal distance between lines 1 and 2 is a measure of the likely distance required for a detonation to form. Note that as the initial pressure falls to a few bar the curves become closer. This is because such a pressure represents a condition when only deflagrations are possible.

5.9 Influence of initial temperature and pressure of the medium on run-up distances

There are little experimental data available on the effect of initial pressure [280] and even less on the influence of initial temperature on the distance necessary for the formation of steadily-propagating detonation waves. A study of the effects of pressure on stoichiometric mixtures of oxygen and hydrogen and on a $C_2H_2 + 2.5O_2 + 4N_2$ mixture showed that for the former mixture the induction length, 0.7 m at 1 bar, was halved when the pressure was increased to 5 bar. Increasing the pressure of the mixture of acetylene, oxygen and nitrogen had an even more pronounced effect [281]. In a 16 mm diameter tube an increase from one to four bar resulted in the run-up distance falling from 0.52 to 0.18 m.

Figure 5.13 shows experimental results for the dependence of X_d on both initial temperature and pressure of the mixture [177], confirming the earlier result that X_d decreases with increasing pressure (p_o) [140], and suggesting that a law of the form

$$X_d = \frac{k}{(p_o)^m} \qquad (5.25)$$

with k = constant and $0.4 < m < 0.8$ may be appropriate. The results for fuels which decompose in the absence of oxygen are more difficult to summarize concisely. For pure acetylene, they exhibit considerable scatter and Fig. 5.12 suggests that X_d may well be independent of pressure. However, it has been suggested that detonations in hydrogen peroxide can be described by Equation 5.25 with $m = 0.5$ [140].

It is interesting to note that there is no obvious reason for the strong influence of pressure in reducing X_d in the theoretical analysis of accelerating flames expressed by Equations 5.22 and 5.23. In general, pressure increases in the range of 0.1 to 5 bar should have relatively minor effects on S_u and ϵ and consequently on g_f. Only for mixtures with relatively high values of laminar burning velocities, fuels such as hydrogen and acetylene, does S_u increase with increasing pressure, and the expansion ratio might be expected to decrease with increasing pressure of the mixture. It is conceivable that the initial pressure of the mixture affects the growth of turbulence, modifying the simple relationship between S_u and S_t expressed in Equation 5.24.

The dependence of X_d on the initial temperature of stoichiometric oxy-hydrogen mixtures has been found to increase from $X_d = 0.6$ m at 288 K to $X_d = 0.73$ m at 398 K and $X_d > 1$ m or total suppression of the detonation at $T > 573$ K [282]. However, the results shown in Fig. 5.13 [177] suggest that any change in X_d for a rise in temperature of 160 K of a $1.5\,H_2 + O_2$ mixture is within the experimental scatter. An appeal to our analysis of distances for shock formation is of little avail. Thus, the initial temperature will influence both S_u and ϵ and consequently g_f; the increased temperature of the unburnt mixture also raises the speed of sound in the unburnt mixture (approximately by 50% for a rise in 160 K in the $1.5\,H_2 + O_2$ mixture) and should result in an increase in X_d. However, this may well be countered by the increase in S_u and ϵ at elevated temperatures producing a higher value of g_f.

5.10 Influence of diameter of pipeline on run-up distances

It would be injudicious to suggest that the mechanisms which control the acceleration of flames in the large diameters of pipelines, typical of chemical

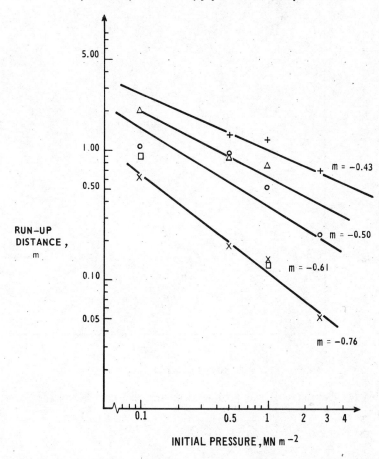

Figure 5.13 Influence of initial pressure and temperature on run-up distances in various fuel–oxygen mixtures [172, 177]. □ = $1.5H_2 + O_2$, 473 K; × = $1.5H_2 + O_2$, 311 K; △ = $H_2 + N_2O$, 311 K; ○ = $CH_4 + 5.67 O_2$, 313 K; + = $2CO + O_2$, 313 K.

plant, are similar to those operating in pipes with $d \leq 50$ mm. For instance, even under idealized conditions, the effects of viscous drag at the wall of tubes of large diameter in lowering the acceleration of a flame will be greatly reduced. Again, closure of the turbulent boundary layer behind any shock propagating into the unreacted medium will be delayed in tubes of large diameter. It is also important to consider the possibilities of effects arising from stratification of mixtures in large diameter pipes and from the likely rougher surface finishes of such pipes.

Available experimental data on the effects of diameter of a pipeline on X_d are somewhat confusing and could well involve the effects of fortuitous changes in another variable, such as the smoothness of the wall. There are

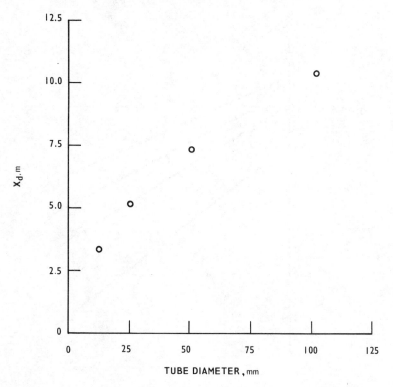

Figure 5.14   Dependence of run-up distance on tube diameter in mixtures of town gas and air [47].

some indications of a change in the mechanism controlling the acceleration of the flame as the bore of the pipe is increased. For small bore pipelines, there is convincing evidence for a relationship between X_d and the square root of the diameter. Figure 5.14 illustrates results for a stoichiometric mixture of town gas with air in pipes $d \leq 102$ mm [47]. The best fit to these results is given by $X_d = Kd^{0.44}$, where K is a constant. A similar law, $X_d = 0.47 \sqrt{d}$, has been reported for mixtures of various fuels with oxygen and nitrogen in pipes of $d \leq 51$ mm [283]. There are two further sets of conflicting data for tubes of $d \leq 51$ mm: (1) Bollinger *et al.* [172, 177, 274], who studied a range of fuels and oxidants, report that only for fuel-rich mixtures of hydrogen and oxidant does pipe diameter affect run-up distances; (2) a study of detonations in mixtures of carbon disulphide and oxygen [284] suggests a direct dependence of X_d on diameter – however, there is general agreement on an $X_d = Kd$ relationship for pipelines of large diameter. This has been found to be applicable to mixtures of hydrogen, methane, nitrogen and nitrogen oxide in pipes of $50 \leq d \leq 500$ mm [285], mixtures of both methane and hydrogen with air in pipes of $d \leq 400$ mm [286] and mixtures of both propane and ethylene with air in pipes of similar bore [275].

There has been only limited progress in attempts to predict the influence of the diameter of pipelines on induction distances for the generation of detonation. For instance, it has been suggested that, for particulate suspensions, it may be related to the closure of the boundary layer behind the shock formed by an accelerating flame [276]. A simplified law describing the growth in thickness of a turbulent boundary layer, δ, with distance behind a shock, X, is [287]

$$\delta = 0.22 X^{0.8} (\mu/\rho_o)^{0.2} \tag{5.26}$$

where μ is the viscosity of the medium behind the shock and ρ_o the density ahead of the shock. With $\delta = 0.5d$ Equation 5.26 results in

$$X_d = \frac{d^{1.25}}{0.36(\mu/\rho_o)} \tag{5.27}$$

in approximate accord with the experimental results obtained in large tubes. Evidently, much more experimental work is required to resolve the question of a possible change in mechanism with increasing diameter of pipe and the possible effects of the nature of the detonable medium on such a change. The need for such work is reinforced by the observation that the velocity of a steadily-propagating wave in mixtures of fuel and air approximately doubles when the diameter of the tube is increased from 13 to 51 mm (Fig. 5.14), indicating the desirability of extending the analysis to include an energy-loss term when describing the formation of a detonation in pipes with $d < 50$ mm [47].

5.11 Effect of additives on pre-detonation distances

The pronounced effect of departures from stoichiometry in increasing run-up distances was discussed in Section 5.8. Only a limited amount of information is available on additives other than the fuel and oxidant. The sole systematic examination of the influence of a variety of additives on pre-detonation distances was carried out in spark-ignited mixtures of acetylene and oxygen and of pentane and oxygen [288]. The mixtures were contained at atmospheric pressure in glass tubes of 9 mm internal diameter. The effects of increasing dilution of a stoichiometric oxy-acetylene mixture are illustrated in Fig. 5.15. Although the value for the mixture in the absence of an additive was not measured, about 0.05 m is a reasonable estimate [177]. Additives evidently exert a strong effect on pre-detonation distances, although it is not clear whether this is due to their reducing the laminar burning velocity or the temperature of the shocked flow for a given velocity of flame, or (as more likely) by a combination of both.

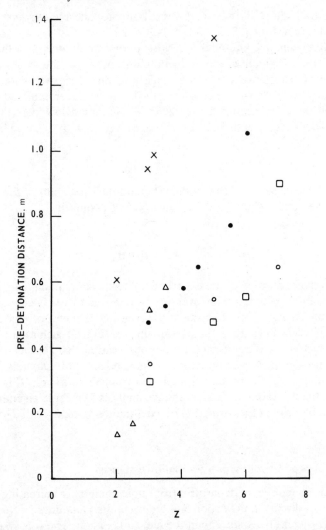

Figure 5.15 Influence of additives on run-up distances in $C_2H_2 + 2.5O_2 + ZM$ mixtures (after Egerton and Gates [288]). $\times$, M = CO_2; $\bullet$, M = N_2; $\bigcirc$, M = Ar; $\triangle$, M = C_2H_2; $\square$, M = O_2.

Certainly, thermal effects are important: additives such as carbon dioxide, which result in low temperatures of burnt gases and shocked flow, are the most effective in inhibiting the formation of the front. Pentane is particularly effective in this respect. However, there appear to be anomalies at low dilutions, when the effects of oxygen, fuel and argon are closely comparable. The additions of between 0.5 and 1.0% of the anti-knocks tetraethyl lead and diethyl selenide, were found to produce chemical effects reducing pre-detonation distances in mixtures diluted with nitrogen, but not with carbon dioxide. Since mixtures of tetraethyl lead and oxygen are known to be detonable [182], it may be that the result pertained to an initial detonation fuelled by the anti-knock itself.

5.12 Effects of surface roughness and obstacles on acceleration of confined flames

The pronounced influence of turbulence in promoting acceleration of flames has been noted in previous sections. It has proved extremely difficult to produce a quantitative relationship between turbulence and the roughness of pipe surface covering the range of surface finishes likely to occur in chemical plant. Some appreciation of the probable magnitude of such effects can be gained from the widely-appreciated reduction in X_d brought about by the introduction of a wire spiral into a pipeline. Typically a spiral of some ten turns of wire 1 mm in diameter at a pitch of about 5 mm can produce a reduction of a factor of ≤ 10 in tubes of diameter $10 < d < 100$ mm. Such a dramatic reduction in X_d suggests that the spiral must be effective in not only the initial phase of acceleration of the flame, but also the period following the formation of an initial shock. In this stage, partial reflections of the shock could promote the ignition of a second flame closer to the leading wave, resulting in the transition to detonation [200]. Recent work on the processes whereby arrays of obstacles of similar or slightly larger dimensions than those typical of Shchelkin spirals accelerate cylindrically-expanding flames has shown that the regularity of spacing may be important [289–291]. Thus the acceleration, following the introduction of a single obstacle, was found to decay, producing a flame travelling at the normal velocity at some distance downstream. Only when a number of regularly-placed obstacles were present was their effect cumulative: the delayed ignition of the mixture in the wake of each obstacle played the principal role in the acceleration of the flame.

Some generalizations about the possible effects of surface finishes likely to be encountered in chemical plant may be helpful. For instance, it is worth bearing in mind that regular undulations are frequently produced in deposits of dusts on the bottom of long, straight runs of pipelines through which dusts are conveyed pneumatically. Their significance may be reduced by the fact that the velocity of the conveying airstream is frequently sufficiently high for the flow to be fully turbulent. Corrugated expansion bellows are occasionally used in plant, but their similarity to Shchelkin spirals renders their use in plant containing flammable media inadvisable. The practice of fabricating bends in pipelines of mild steel from angled sections of straight pipelines is also unsuitable, unless appropriate precautions are taken with the internal welds. When estimating, from data obtained from experimental apparatus, available distances for the injection of a flame inhibitor or the position at which internal stresses appropriate to a C–J wave are first formed, it is generally reasonable to divide such values of X_d by two, to allow for the rougher internal finishes of pipelines in industrial plant. However, when considering the possibility of pressure piling (discussed in Section 5.13), the longer the induction distance, the greater is the possibility of its occurrence. Consequently, some caution must be exercised when applying an arbitrary correction factor.

5.13 Pressure piling (cascading)

When the distance required for a detonation to form is comparable with the length of installed pipeline, it is possible that the wave forms in an already compressed medium. Consequently, internal stresses can be produced which are well in excess of that generated by a C–J wave travelling in the medium at its original pressure. Since the probability of pressure piling increases with increasing run-up distance, it is convenient to discuss it at this stage. Although its potential for damage has long been recognized, well-authenticated examples in either experimental apparatus or industrial explosions are difficult to find [292]. It has most frequently been considered in terms of detonations in pure acetylene, but has also been recognized as a possibility in explosions transmitted through a pipeline connecting two vessels, with both vessels and pipeline filled by a mixture of fuel and oxidant [293].

The process is most readily visualized in terms of a pipeline closed at the end distant from the source of ignition or with a reactor vessel there. As the flame accelerates away from the igniter a pressure gradient builds up in the pipeline. A shock may either be produced in the flow propagating towards the closed end or, following the reflection and coalescence of pressure waves from the closed end, as a wave propagating back towards the igniter. The highest internal pressures are likely to be generated in the latter case, when the reflected shock transforms into a detonation. The magnification factor will vary along the length of the pipeline on account of the pressure gradient with the highest factor occurring close to the flame front. As an approximate guideline the factor is likely to be between two and five.

The situation when a reactor vessel is connected to the end of the pipeline is more complex, as a change in area of confinement will generally be present. Such a change will not have a significant effect on the early stages of pressurization, when the rates of rise in pressure are low. It will, however, play an important role in attenuating any shock [294, 295] or detonation [35, 89] travelling into the vessel. The attenuation of detonations in expansions in area is dealt with in detail in Chapter 6. At this stage it is sufficient to note that a portion of the original detonation shock propagates for some distance into the larger vessel before the expansion waves meet at the axis of symmetry. A decreasing area of high pressure can continue to exist for up to ten diameters in the reactor vessel.

Closely related to these forms of pressure piling are the effects of the various forms of wave interactions associated with the formation of a forward-

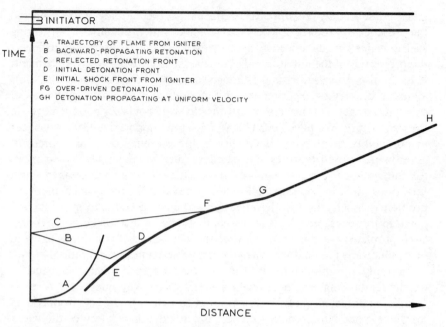

Figure 5.16   Generation of high pressures near to the closed ignition end, as reflected retonation and incident detonation coalesce.

facing detonation wave. It has been widely recognized that anomalously high pressures can be developed over short distances close to the plane at which a detonation is formed. A particularly well-documented example is that on the formation of detonations in mixtures of ammonia and nitrous oxide in tubes of 85 mm diameter [161]. The generation of high pressures can be accounted for in terms of Fig. 5.16. At the instant the forward-facing detonation is formed a retonation wave is also created, and this travels back through the burnt mixture towards the closed end from which it reflects. On account of the high speed of sound in the reacted mixture, the reflected retonation overtakes the detonation. For a short distance, prior to attenuation by the following expansion fan, the combined front is strongly overdriven. The magnitude of the anomalous stresses and the length of pipeline over which they exist varies with the nature of the medium, the dimensions of the containment and the position of the initiator relative to the closed end of the tube. Experimental evidence suggests that magnification factors of up to three, stretching over distances of up to 30 diameters are possible.

5.14 Concluding remarks

Key questions in an analysis of risk from a plant processing exothermally-reacting media concern the probability of a detonation occurring, and how this is influenced by the properties of the media, the initiator, its position and the presence or absence of a degree of confinement. Difficulties in answering such questions are enhanced by the clear evidence for the interrelationships of the properties of the initiator and of the media to the degree of confinement. It is not altogether surprising, although somewhat disappointing, that, after almost a century of experimental and theoretical work on the initiation of detonations, general answers to such questions are not likely to be achieved in the near future. We have been able to draw attention to significant advances in our ability to predict detonability in the presence of weak sources of ignition in confined mixtures of fuel and oxidant, and to possible correlations for confined aerosols and clouds of dusts. There remain wide areas in which little or no directly-applicable information is available; for instance, there are problems associated with the effect of additives in confined systems, and much more severe problems in the general area of unconfined detonations. Such problems are compounded when the wide range of conditions likely to be produced by the malfunction of plant are taken into consideration.

Presently, it is difficult to pinpoint a particular area in which an advance in our understanding would result in answers to the key questions. A more complete appreciation of the spontaneous growth of transverse fronts on an incipient spherical detonation could allow for the application of the wider range of data available on confined fronts. This would represent a considerable gain, in that experiments on spherical waves are both time-consuming and expensive. Further work concentrated on initiation in marginally-detonable media is obviously desirable, in that these are the most likely to occur in practice. Finally, and possibly of greatest import, is a thorough study of the effects of inhomogeneities in composition of the medium, since these are likely to be a common feature of confined and unconfined detonations.

Even after gaining these objectives a severe problem remains in relating the information to the range of conditions likely to be encountered following a fault in a plant. Their importance is best illustrated by an example – consider a confined detonation initiated in a pocket of fuel-rich mixture of hydrocarbon and oxidant and propagating into a composition gradient which falls to below the normal fuel-lean limit of detonability. Initiation in successive layers occurs via a leading front of higher than the C–J velocity appropriate to that layer. It is quite conceivable that initiation by an overdriven wave of this type could lead to a widening of the effective limits. The converse situation is also possible, in which there is an underdriven wave in the initiator, perhaps resulting in a narrowing of effective limits. In order to produce reliable assessments of the dangers of a detonation, it may be necessary to specify the most probable locations of the source and the composition gradients which result in significant changes in the C–J velocity. This may be possible in the case of vapour clouds, where a drop in concentration of fuel with increasing distance from the leak can be anticipated, but such well-defined conditions are the exception rather than the rule.

Presently, the best advice which can be given for the conservative design of plant containing mixtures within pressure and composition limits of flammability is that the possibility of a detonation should be considered. Only when the length of pipelines in such plant is considerably below the theoretical run-up distance and the possibility of the occurrence of any ignition source of energy greater than the minimum ignition energy (which can be as low as a few millijoules) can be excluded, is it possible to rule out the possibility of a detonation. These are particularly stringent conditions for aerosols and dust clouds where the possibility of static charging is always present. There are obvious dangers in attempting to offer such specific suggestions when considering the possibility of unconfined detonations, especially in terms of local formation of a front within the cloud. Investigations of well documented and truly unconfined cloud explosions point to the requirement of extensive clouds, of diameters say 50 m or more, and suggest the need for initiators with energies of some orders of magnitude greater than the minimum ignition energy.

6

Interaction of a detonation with confinement

6.1 Introductory remarks

Although a limited number of the qualitative aspects of the interaction of detonations with certain types of change in confinement have been studied, no general theoretical treatment has emerged. Indeed, some of the stochastic properties of detonation waves indicate that such a development is unlikely [206, 207, 296]. It may be helpful to outline some of the current problems in formulating such an analysis. In order to do so, it is necessary to appeal extensively to experimental and theoretical work on planar shock waves in non-reactive media. However, as a recent review makes clear [297], even with this simplification it is only possible to deal comprehensively with the diffraction of a shock by an isolated wall. The interactions between the wave systems generated at further walls in the vicinity of the first with those set up by diffraction at the first are so complex that, at best, it is only possible to consider averaged effects.

The problem is compounded by the fact that, depending on the Mach number of the incident shock and the angle of inclination of the wall, a transition in the process of diffraction occurs. Thus, at small angles of inclination, the incident front suffers a Mach reflection, as described in terms of the transverse fronts on a detonation wave in Chapter 1. The configuration of triple shocks consists of the Mach stem OM, the incident front OI and the reflected shock wave OR, with gas treated by the Mach stem divided from that treated by the incident and reflected waves by the slipstream OS (Fig. 1.3), across which the pressure is constant. As the angle of the wedge is increased a change to regular reflection occurs, when the Mach stem disappears and the gas is treated by both incident (IO) and reflected (OR) shocks. Normal reflection, when the planar shock encounters a wall of angle 90° is thus a limiting case of regular reflection. The existence of two forms of reflection at surfaces with positive angles of inclination has led to the development and continued use of two separate theories of shock diffraction, the Chester–

Chisnell–Whitham (CCW) analysis [298–300] and the standard two-shock theory [301], both having advantages in certain situations. In particular, CCW theory can readily be applied to walls with both negative and positive angles of inclination. As such it is of more general applicability. In addition, it combines the merits of simplicity in use with an acceptable accuracy in predicting the averaged properties of the diffracted wave. Thus, CCW theory is extensively used throughout this chapter and the somewhat sparse experimental evidence justifying its application to detonation waves, especially non-steady and non-planar ones, emphasized.

For the purposes of design of plant, the theoretical treatment should ideally result in accurate predictions of the peak local pressure, its variation with time and location. In addition, accurate descriptions of the variation in profile of the leading shock during the process of diffraction should allow assessments of the pressure generated at the surface of any obstruction encountered by the diffracting shock. As will become increasingly clear, much further work is required in order to meet these objectives. On the more positive side however, there is a growing understanding of the mechanisms whereby changes in the shape of confinement result in properties of the front varying widely from those predicted by unidimensional theories of detonation waves.

There are problems in presenting information on the interactions of detonations with surfaces in the most readily utilizable fashion. We have chosen to start with isolated expansive corners, partly on account of the fact that the interactions of shocks and detonations with a wall of negative angle of inclination ($\theta_w < 0$) have been most widely studied, and partly on account of their practical implications, both in terms of quenching and of initiation of expanding detonations. This results in the natural introduction of CCW theory. Section 6.3 extends this to walls $0 < \theta_w < \theta_{crit}$, where θ_{crit} is the angle of inclination at which the transition to regular reflection takes place. In the following section, two-shock theory is described and applied to regular reflection with walls of $\theta_{crit} < \theta_w < 90°$. Section 6.5 is devoted to normal reflection. The rudimentary treatments given in Sections 6.3–6.5 are for planar fronts. Presently, it is only possible to call attention to the likely differences in behaviour between planar and curved fronts of unconfined detonations and of those propagating through marginally-detonable media. However, we do describe methods for taking into account the change in specific heat ratio across the fronts, in order to avoid the common but erroneous overestimate of peak pressures based on non-reactive shock theory. Section 6.6 deals with the most widely-studied change in confinement, an abrupt area change [35, 89]. In this and the following section on bends and junctions (Section 6.7), we have extrapolated from the wave systems produced at isolated walls to the probable interactions between them, which can either result in quenching or the eventual re-establishment of a steady detonation. On account of the paucity of data on detonations, much of this extrapolation is perforce based on the interactions of planar shocks in non-reactive media. However, application of data of shock waves to reactive media does lead to a number of suggestions about features of design which minimize the asymmetrical nature of local pressure histories and possibly reduce the amplitude of local peaks in pressure.

Two further related topics merit inclusion in this chapter. The first concerns the effects of an inert and compressible boundary layer in attenuating the velocity of a detonation propagating through an inner core of the explosive mixture. It may be possible in a limited number of practical situations to make use of such an effect to protect particularly vulnerable portions of plant. The other topic is the refraction, resulting from changes in temperature or composition of the medium, of a detonation wave propagating through a gradient of sound speed. Such effects are of particular relevance to the effects of a detonation in a large cloud of vapour in which such gradients are likely to occur.

6.2 Diffraction at an isolated wall, $\theta_w < 0°$

It is necessary to start with an outline of the process of the diffraction of a planar shock at an isolated wall before going on to consider the additional complexities associated with the diffraction of a planar detonation front. Figure 6.1 is a sketch of such a front, Mach number M_o, propagating around a wall where $\theta_w < 0°$. Centred on the corner, O, is a Prandtl–Meyer expansion fan SOT, the head of which (OS) propagates into the flow at an angle m_o, to an extension of the wall and defines the unattenuated portion of the incident front SR. The attenuating front ST is joined to a straight wall shock, propagating orthogonally along the corner wall at a Mach number $M_w < M_o$. The flow behind SR is parallel to the direction in which the front SR propagates and m_o is given by

$$\arctan^2 m_o = \frac{(\gamma - 1)(M_o^2 - 1)[M_o^2 + 2/(\gamma - 1)]}{(\gamma + 1)M_o^4} \tag{6.1}$$

and somewhat less accurately by CCW theory as

$$\arctan m_o = \frac{1}{M_o}\left(\frac{M_o^2 - 1}{n}\right)^{0.5} \tag{6.2}$$

where $n = 2/K(M_o)$ where K is a constant and n is thus a slowly varying function of M_o. Table 6.1 gives the values of n calculated for strong shocks

Table 6.1 Calculated values of n for strong shocks and detonations.

γ	1.667	1.400	1.200
n	4.4361	5.0743	6.1311

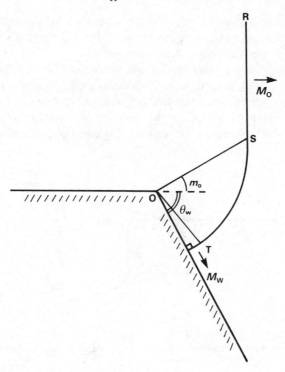

Figure 6.1   Diffraction of a shock at a wall $\theta_w < 0°$.

$(M_o \rightarrow \infty)$ in media of different ratios of specific heats. For $M_o \geq 4.5$, typical of C–J velocities of detonations, the simpler Equation 6.2 is adequate, since the approximation on which it is based $n \neq f(M)$ becomes fully justifiable.

Consider now a detonation travelling through a divergent nozzle. In the following sections, it will be shown that M_w decreases for increasingly negative values of θ_w. For low values of M_w, temperatures and densities, even behind the curved portion of the front TS, are insufficient for ignition to occur, behind a transverse front. Only when the interaction of a transverse front is sufficiently strong to result in temperatures and densities comparable with those behind a C–J front can the detonation re-establish itself. Thus, whether the detonation is quenched or not depends on the inclination of the walls and the properties of the transverse fronts, namely their spacing and strengths. Unfortunately, there is little prospect of developing a general theory to account fully for the processes involved. This becomes clear for an examination of the case of a single-headed detonation when there is no way of predicting the position of the transverse front as the detonation enters the expansion, and thus of estimating the changes in its associated flow field during its interactions in the expansion fan and at the wall [296]. The non-planarity of detonation fronts in marginally-detonable media presents a further problem; estimates of m_o and M_w are based on the assumption that the flow behind the unattenuated portion of the front is parallel to the axis of symmetry. This does not apply to marginal waves.

It is possible to give an outline of the processes involved, based on the diffraction of a non-reactive wave. The distance along a divergent nozzle at which such a wave becomes completely curved, x, is shown in Fig. 6.2 to be given by $x = r/\tan m_o$, where r is the radius or half-height of the inlet. The interactions which result in a constant velocity of propagation over the entire

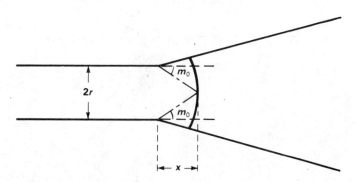

Figure 6.2   Attenuation of a planar shock in a gradually-divergent channel.

periphery of the front of M_w are generally complete in a further axial distance of $2x$. This velocity can be estimated relatively simply using CCW theory. Its basic equation, relating the change in area of the front, brought about by a wall of inclination θ_w with change in Mach number dM is

$$\theta_w = \int_{M_o}^{M_w} \left[\frac{n}{M^2 - 1} \right]^{0.5} dM \qquad (6.3)$$

Integrating with the boundary condition $\theta_w = 0$, $M = M_{CJ}$ results in

$$\frac{M_w}{M_{CJ}} = \frac{1}{2M_{CJ}} [\{M_{CJ} + \sqrt{(M_{CJ}^2 - 1)}\} \exp{(\theta_w/\sqrt{n})}$$
$$+ \{M_{CJ} + \sqrt{(M_{CJ}^2 - 1)}\} \exp{(\theta_w/\sqrt{n})^{-1}}] \qquad (6.4)$$

Since $M_{CJ}^2 \gg 1$ the approximate solution

$$\frac{M_w}{M_{CJ}} = \exp{(\theta_w/\sqrt{n})} \qquad (6.5)$$

is generally of sufficient accuracy. Table 6.2 shows values of M_w/M_{CJ} calculated from Equation 6.5 for media of various ratios of specific heats. It is possible to make an approximate estimate of the value of M_w at which

Table 6.2 Dependence of M_w/M_{CJ} on θ_w.

θ_w (degrees)	-10	-20	-30	-40	-50	-60	-70	-80	-90
$M_w/M_{CJ}, \gamma = 1.67$	.92	.83	.78	.72	.66	.61	.56	.52	.47
$M_w/M_{CJ}, \gamma = 1.4$	.93	.84	.79	.73	.68	.63	.58	.54	.50
$M_w/M_{CJ}, \gamma = 1.2$	.93	.85	.81	.75	.70	.66	.61	.58	.53

quenching of the reaction fronts behind transverse shocks occurs, by assuming that the interactions of transverse fronts with the walls are always sufficiently weak for reignition not to occur, and then using data on the failure processes within a single detonation cell. From these it is reasonable to suggest that failure occurs with $M_w/M_{CJ} \sim 0.6$ in a gradual expansion, perhaps increasing to $M_w/M_{CJ} \sim 0.8$ in an abrupt expansion [302]. Taking the latter gives $\theta_w = -29°$ in a medium of $\gamma = 1.4$.

In nozzles with angles of divergence less than this, a curved but steady front with approximately the C–J velocity should be produced, provided that at least one transverse front travels into the expansion region before the heads of the fan meet at the axis of symmetry. Since the velocity of the transverse fronts is approximately sonic, this proviso can be expressed in terms of the transit time of a transverse front S/a_{CJ} being less than the time required for the crossing of the heads of the expansion fan, so that

$$S/r = \frac{a_{CJ}}{a_o M_{CJ} \tan m_o} \qquad (6.6)$$

Substituting values typical of a detonation wave in Equation 6.6, $a_{CJ}/a_o \sim 3$, $M_{CJ} \sim 6$ and $m_o = 24°$, suggests that there should be at least two transverse fronts on the incident wave in order for a steady detonation to be produced.

To date there have been too few experimental studies to confirm such theories. Early experiments, [303, 304] reviewed by Bazhenova *et al.* [303], were carried out with stoichiometric mixtures of methane with oxygen at atmospheric pressure and with $\theta_w \le -65°$. With such an angle the process of re-establishment may correspond more closely with those in an abrupt expansion, in which it is controlled by the conditions in the flow field close to the head of the expansion fan, rather than those behind the wall shock. However, these experiments did show that, as with non-reactive shocks, the process of diffraction is self-similar i.e. the curvature of the front is preserved throughout the process, justifying the application of CCW theory. Furthermore, an incident front with closely-spaced transverse fronts was observed to fail, in accord with the present analysis, at about $\theta_w = -65°$. Thus, for a C–J detonation in $CH_4 + 2O_2$ propagating through a divergence of $\theta_w = -65°$, Equation 6.5 gives $M_w/M_{CJ} \sim 0.6$, the failure criterion based on observations of a single cell.

Some features of the interaction of detonations which have been observed in the gradually divergent sections of convergent–divergent nozzles have still to be explained. Thus, an interferometric study of a detonation travelling through a nozzle with small but unspecified angle of divergence clearly demonstrated the disappearance of transverse waves and consequent quenching [305]. However, a further study employing an 'open-shutter' camera technique showed little change in the structure of a front in either the divergent or convergent sections of a nozzle of $\theta_w = \pm 16°$ [306]. This led to the suggestion that only detonations with a single transverse wave are quenched in gradually divergent nozzles. There must be some doubt as to the sensitivity of the open-shutter technique, since it failed to reveal the decrease in spacing of transverse fronts at the start of the convergent section. The increase in the number of transverse waves at similar wall angles has been well established by a number of workers using a variety of experimental techniques [33]. Finally, there is some experimental evidence indicating that leading detonation fronts attenuate somewhat more rapidly than non-reactive shocks in gradual divergences [91, 307]. The balance of available experimental evidence suggests that even multi-headed detonation fronts may be quenched in gradually divergent nozzles.

The local wall pressure naturally depends on whether and at what position a curved detonation front is established downstream of the divergence. Following re-establishment, the normal considerations described in Chapter 2 are applicable. There have been no experimental measurements of the local pressures generated at a divergent wall by a diffracting detonation. For the case of a failing front, the pressure should fall from an approximate value corresponding with a non-reactive shock at the wall (with M_w given by Equation 6.5) to the value appropriate to a steady detonation at the position of the head of the expansion fan. On account of the transverse fronts propagating into the decaying zone, the local pressures will be somewhat higher than those predicted by substitution of the relevant Mach number in Equation 6.3. An alternative approach, making due allowance for this, is to base designs on peak pressures corresponding with a steady detonation front until the head of the expansion has crossed the complete periphery of the incident wave. The strength of the leading front of a failed detonation (downstream of this position) can then be calculated from the area ratio technique described in Section 6.3. There is no information available on the way in which the pressure versus time characteristics of the wave change during the transition process. Although the empirical laws relating the location of the C–J plane with dimensions of a detonation cell are essentially those for a planar leading wave, it is necessary to retain them in predicting the shapes of pressure history produced by the curved front and to extrapolate from the properties of a blast front for positions downstream of the point of failure.

6.3 Diffraction at an isolated wall, $0° < \theta_w < \theta_{crit}$

Detailed studies of the diffraction of shocks in non-reactive media on walls of positive angles of inclination have shown that two types of reflection process can occur. As will be shown later, the same is true of detonation waves. However, it will be useful to consider first the simpler case of shocks in non-reactive media outlined in Section 6.1 and shown in Fig. 6.3. At low values of θ_w the incident front IO, Mach number M_o, suffers a Mach reflection forming a Mach stem OM, travelling at right angles to the wall at a constant trajectory χ with a Mach number $M_w > M_o$. It is joined at the triple point O to a

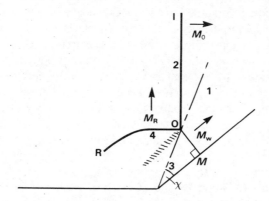

Figure 6.3 Mach reflection with gas in region 2 treated by a front velocity M_0, in region 3 by a front of velocity M_w and in region 4 by fronts of velocity M_0 and M_R.

reflected shock OR. At larger values of θ_w the incident wave undergoes regular reflection, when the flow is rendered parallel to the inclined wall by the reflected wave OR. The critical angle for the transition from Mach to regular reflection θ_{crit} depends on the velocity of the incident front and the ratio of specific heats of the medium.

Although more complex forms of combined Mach and regular reflection can be observed over a narrow range of experimental parameters in non-reactive media [308], they have not as yet been observed with detonations. A comparison of the profiles of the reflected waves produced by the diffraction of a detonation in a stoichiometric mixture of methane and oxygen with those generated by a planar shock of similar velocity in carbon dioxide on a wedge of $\theta_w = 24°$, indicated that the detonation suffered simple Mach reflection, whilst the shock formed a double Mach configuration [304]. This is explicable in terms of the liberation of chemical energy in the flow behind the detonation, which results in flow becoming subsonic. Consequently, complex forms of reflection of detonations should only occur when the leading wave is so strongly overdriven that the flow behind it becomes supersonic. However, in view of the complex double triple-point configurations observed to occur in detonations in mixtures of carbon monoxide and oxygen in straight-walled channels [64], it would be rash to predicate that complex reflections can only occur, providing the leading wave is initially overdriven.

There are two essential differences between the diffraction of non-reactive shocks and detonations. The first of these involves the effects of the collisions of the natural transverse fronts with the reflected wave produced at the inclined wall. The second concerns the effects of the complex flow fields existing behind the incident non-linear detonation. With a linear non-reactive shock diffracting on a wedge, the particle paths are normal to the incident wave and consequently parallel to a linear reflected wave. While it is possible to model some of the effects of divergent particle paths by studying the diffraction of curved blast waves, it is evidently extremely difficult to account for the effects of the non-stationary reaction zones in modifying the flow field. It is therefore not surprising that there is no general theory of reflection of detonation waves by wedges. Intuitively, it might be expected that the theories developed for non-reactive shocks should apply more closely to a detonation with closely-spaced transverse fronts, when non-linearity and divergence of the flow field is minimized. However, it is probable that the poor performance of these theories in areas such as the prediction of θ_{crit} deteriorates further when they are applied to detonations.

In applying the CCW analysis to detonations it should be noted that an integral part, the Chester–Chisnell approximate relationship [299] between area and Mach number of a shock, is expected to be less accurate in describing contracting fronts than it is for expanding waves. Despite this limitation and some uncertainty about its performance in dealing with curved incident fronts, the simplicity and versatility of CCW merits a full description of its application to diffraction of detonations by compressive surfaces. Accepting its limitations, the analysis gives a reasonable estimate of the Mach number of the Mach stem and consequently the pressure behind it and, with somewhat less accuracy, the trajectory of the triple point. The basic equations are (6.7), giving the relationship between the average Mach number of the incident wave M_{CJ} and that of the Mach stem M_{w} in terms of the wall angle θ_{w} and the corresponding areas of front A_{CJ} and A_{w} respectively,

$$\cot \theta_{\text{w}} = \frac{M_{\text{CJ}}}{M_{\text{w}}} \left\{ \frac{1 + A_{\text{w}} M_{\text{w}} / A_{\text{CJ}} M_{\text{CJ}}}{[(1 - M_{\text{CJ}}^2 / M_{\text{w}}^2)(1 - A_{\text{w}}^2 / A_{\text{CJ}}^2)]^{0.5}} \right\} \tag{6.7}$$

and the analogous equation for χ

$$\tan \chi = \frac{A_{\text{w}}}{A_{\text{CJ}}} \left(\frac{1 - M_{\text{CJ}}^2 / M_{\text{w}}^2}{1 - A_{\text{w}}^2 / A_{\text{CJ}}^2} \right)^{0.5} \tag{6.8}$$

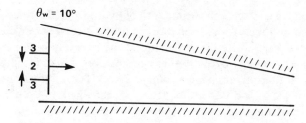

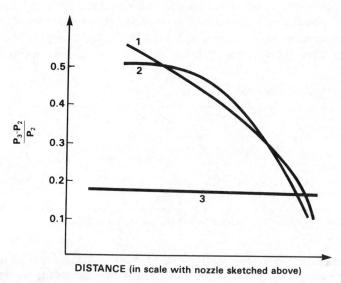

Figure 6.4 Decay in strength of natural transverse fronts on a detonation travelling through a constriction (after Strehlow *et al.* [307]. 1, 2 transverse fronts; 3 wall-generated front.

There have been few systematic studies of the diffraction of detonations on isolated walls with small angles of inclination [33, 91] or in gradually convergent channels [305, 306]. Those which have been carried out have led to apparently conflicting results, probably on account of partly opposing effects of two different phenomena. While theoretical predictions indicate that at the start of the convergence the spacing of the transverse waves should decrease behind the strengthened Mach stem, (as indeed was shown to be the case for an isolated wall, by both smoked-foil and schlieren techniques) [33] the transverse fronts have been found to disappear from a detonation propagating through a convergent channel of similar angle of inclination [305]. The explanation may lie in an energy loss process, weakening the strength of the transverse fronts as the detonation travels through a nozzle. For instance, this might occur during the interaction of the transverse fronts with the boundary layer on the opposite wall. Figure 6.4 [307] illustrates the decay of transverse waves on detonations in a stoichiometric mixture of hydrogen and oxygen diluted with 50% argon, in their propagation through a constriction of one plane wall and one inclined at $\theta_w = 10°$. The strengths of the naturally-occurring transverse fronts 1 and 2 rapidly decay during transmission, whilst the strength of the wall-generated front remains constant at $Z = 3$. The natural transverse fronts are typically damped out in about 10 cell lengths [307]. At this stage an improved performance is to be expected from CCW theory.

Critical wall angles for the transition from Mach to regular reflection on isolated walls have been measured for detonations in four different mixtures [33, 303]. Table 6.3 lists these, their C–J velocities, their ratio of specific heats and the spacing of transverse waves. The CCW treatment implies the existence of a triple shock configuration, so can only lead to an approximate

Table 6.3 Experimental values of critical angles [33, 303].

Mixture	M_{CJ}	S (mm)	γ	θ_{crit}
$C_2H_2 + 2.5O_2 + 8.17$ Ar	5.5	8	1.575	~50°
$2H_2 + O_2 +$ Ar	5.1	6	1.470	$46° < \theta_{crit} < 50°$
$C_2H_2 + 2.5O_2$	7.0	3	1.360	$30° < \theta_{crit} < 38°$
$CH_4 + 2O_2$ [303]	6.3	*	1.370	35°

*Initial pressure of mixture is not quoted by authors, so S cannot be defined.

estimate of θ_{crit}. This is obtained by solving Equations 6.5, 6.7 and 6.8 to give the dependence of χ on θ_w. The results of such calculations for media with $\gamma = 1.67, 1.40$ and 1.20, showing the difficulties in accurately extrapolating to $\chi = 0$ to obtain θ_{crit} are shown in Fig. 6.5. It indicates that, depending on γ for the mixture, defining n as in Equation 6.5, $40° \leq \theta_{crit} \leq 50°$. Standard 2 and 3 shock theories, to be described in the following section, might be expected to perform rather better in predicting θ_{crit}. However, while they give $\theta_{crit} = 50°$ for an argon-diluted stoichiometric oxyacetylene mixture (in close agreement with the measured value), they predict a value of 65° for an argon-diluted stoichiometric oxyhydrogen mixture, for which the experimental value is $48° \pm 2°$. Analyses based on non-reactive shock theories are barely adequate when applied to critical angles; although CCW theory gives a tolerable description of the variations in χ with θ_w for $\theta_w > 30°$. Figure 6.5 also compares experimental values of χ, obtained in heavily diluted stoichiometric oxyacetylene mixtures at different initial pressures, in order to vary the spacing of transverse fronts, with CCW predictions. The experimental results [33] suggest that χ is dependent on spacing, but there is a measure of agreement between theory and experiment for $\theta_w > 10°$.

CCW theory performs much more satisfactorily in describing the enhancement of the wall shock. Figure 6.6 is a comparison of the manner in which

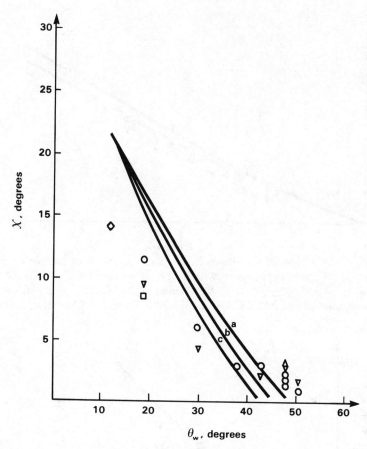

Figure 6.5 Influence of θ_w and γ on the trajectory of triple points in Mach-reflected detonations [33]. a, b and c, CCW theory $\gamma = 1.67$, 1.40 and 1.20 respectively; experimental results 30% $(2C_2H_2 + 5O_2) + 70\%$ Ar. △, 50 torr; ○, 75 torr; ◇, 90 torr; ▽, 100 torr; □, 125 torr.

M_w / M_{CJ} is predicted to vary with θ_w, with experimental values for detonations in a $2H_2 + O_2 + Ar$ mixture and in a stoichiometric oxyacetylene mixture, again diluted with argon [33]. While there is some indication that the measured enhancement depends slightly on the spacing of transverse waves, CCW theory performs in a highly satisfactory fashion. In view of this, it should also produce reliable estimates of the pressure behind the Mach stem, when M_w is substituted in Equation 2.7, for values of $\theta_w < \theta_{crit}$. Figure 6.7 shows this to be the case, when the theory is compared with experimental results for diffracting detonations in stoichiometric oxyacetylene mixtures.

In terms of the normal reflection of a planar detonation front, it is instructive to consider an alternative treatment. Recalling the numbering of

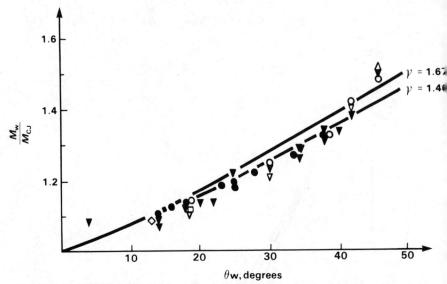

Figure 6.6 CCW analysis of the influence of θ_w and γ on the Mach number of the wall front [33]. Experimental results ▼ schlieren; ● smoked foil $2H_2 + O_2 + Ar$, S = 6 mm, $\gamma = 1.47$, $M_{CJ} = 5.1$; □ S = 4 mm; ▽ S = 5 mm; ◇ S = 6 mm; ○ S = 8 mm, smoked foil, 30% $(2C_2H_2 + 5O_2) + 70\%$ Ar, $M_{CJ} = 5.5$ and $\gamma = 1.44$.

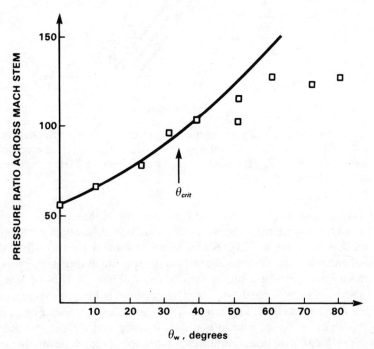

Figure 6.7 CCW analysis of dependence of pressure ratio across Mach stem on θ_w [33]. □, experimental results $2C_2H_2 + 5O_2$, S = 3 mm, $\gamma = 1.36$ and $M_{CJ} = 7.0$.

the regions of gas treated by the various waves shown in Fig. 6.3 and that $p_4 = p_3$, the pressure ratio across the reflected wave p_4/p_2 close to the triple point (where it is reasonable to assume that γ remains constant) is given by

$$\frac{p_4}{p_2} = \frac{p_1}{p_2}\frac{p_3}{p_1} \qquad (6.9)$$

and p_2/p_1 is a function of M_{CJ}^2, as is p_3/p_1 of M_w^2. Figure 6.8 depicts how the pressure ratio across the reflected wave varies with θ_w, with the full line changing to a dashed one at the critical wall angle. The extrapolation of theory to $\theta_w = 90°$ suggests that the pressure ratio at $\theta_w = 90°$ should not exceed 3.5. Included in Fig. 6.8 are experimental results for the variation in p_4/p_2 with θ_w for detonations in $2C_2H_2 + 5O_2$ and $2H_2 + O_2 + Ar$ mixtures [33], together with the mean of experimental measurements on the strength of the normally-reflected wave in stoichiometric oxyhydrogen mixtures over a wide range of initial pressures [16, 309]. There are a number of features to note. Firstly, as might be expected from the performance of CCW theory in predicting the velocity of the Mach stem, the theoretical strengths of the reflected wave for $\theta_w < \theta_{crit}$ are in reasonable agreement with those measured. Indeed, they

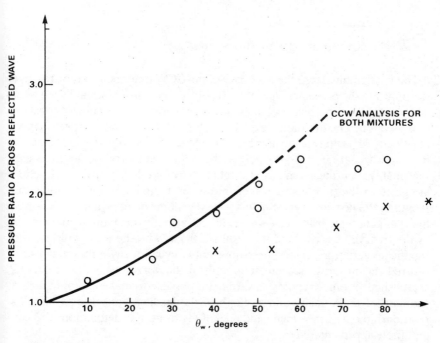

Figure 6.8 Effect of θ_w on strength of reflected waves [33]. $\bigcirc$, $2C_2H_2 + 5O_2$, $\gamma = 1.36$, $M_{CJ} = 7.0$, $S = 3$ mm; $\times$, $2H_2 + O_2 + Ar$, $\gamma = 1.47$, $M_{CJ} = 5.1$, $S = 6.5$ mm; $*2H_2 + O_2$ [16].

model particularly well the behaviour of detonations in stoichiometric oxy-acetylene mixtures, in which the experimental measurements may be some-what more accurate. Secondly, the strength of the reflected wave remains approximately constant for $\theta_w > \theta_{crit}$, suggesting that normally-reflected waves in oxyacetylene mixtures should have a strength of about 2.2 and in oxyhydrogen mixtures about 1.9. This is well below the strength of waves produced by reflection of strong planar shocks in non-reactive media of $\gamma = 1.4$, which may have a strength of up to 8. The explanation of this reduction lies in the effects of the addition of energy in the reaction zones and the change in γ therein, and is dealt with in detail in Section 6.4.

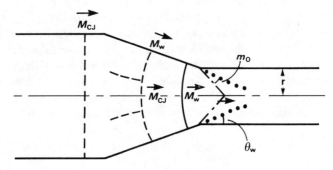

Figure 6.9   Recovery of a C–J front in a contraction.

Having demonstrated the adequacy of the CCW treatment, it is instructive to apply it to the processes whereby a steady detonation is re-established after its propagation through a gradually convergent nozzle in a section of constant cross-section. The situation is sketched in Fig. 6.9 with an incident detonation of velocity M_{CJ} entering the nozzle and the Mach stems formed at the entrance moving with a trajectory χ to meet at the axis of symmetry. Up to this stage, reasonably accurate estimates of local pressures produced by the diffraction are given by the treatment outlined. However, there is a problem should the length of the nozzle exceed that associated with the meeting and reflection of the wall-generated transverse waves. In such a nozzle, the mutual interactions of the transverse waves and the resultant fronts with the walls will result in significant variations in local pressures, until a cylindrically contracting front, centred on the projected meeting point of the nozzle walls at the axis, is established. From this point onwards, it is possible to make an approximate estimate of the velocity and strength of the leading front using Chisnell's relationship between velocity and area of the front. For detonations this can be simply approximated to

$$\frac{A}{A_{CJ}} = \left[\frac{M_{CJ}}{M} \right]^n \tag{6.10}$$

where A is the area of the cylindrical front, A_{CJ} the area of the inlet channel and M the Mach number of the detonation, when its area has shrunk to A. On account of instabilities which arise in imploding shocks, such an analysis must be regarded as a rough approximation. When an overdriven detonation of velocity M_w enters the exit it experiences an expansion, so that Equation 6.11 applies, and gives the distance x at which the heads of the expansion fan meet at the axis thus

$$\frac{x}{r} = \operatorname{arccot}(\theta_w + m_o) \tag{6.11}$$

The process of attenuation across the complete periphery of the detonation to produce a C–J detonation should then be complete within a distance of about $5x$.

The earlier parts of this section showed that it was possible to estimate with reasonable accuracy the observed amplitudes of the initial pressure peaks produced by a detonation diffracting on shallow wedges. However, the same is not true of the subsequent profile of local pressure histories; neither are any significant experimental data available. Some caution must be exercised in extrapolating the relationship between cell size and hydrodynamic thickness developed for a steady wave to a diffracting front. A sketch of a soot track record of a detonation in a stoichiometric oxyacetylene mixture diluted with argon on a 18.5° wedge, Fig. 6.10, shows the random nature of the structure produced behind the triple point [33]. The anticipated increase in density in writing behind the wall-induced transverse wave is evident, indicating a shortening in the duration of peak pressure in the diffracted front compared with a steady front. However, there are evidently wide local variations in the

INCIDENT DETONATION WAVE

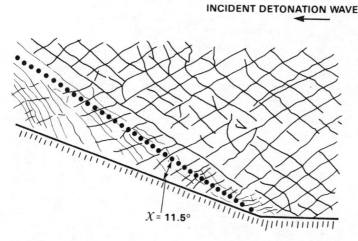

$X = 11.5°$

Figure 6.10 Cellular structure produced by $30\% (2C_2H_2 + 5O_2) + 70\%$ Ar detonation diffracting on a wedge $\theta_w = 18.5°$ [33]; ••• trajectory of triple point.

magnitude of the effect. Furthermore, at the apex of the wedge the random structure penetrates beyond the trajectory of the wall-induced triple point. Evidently there is a need for further work on these aspects.

6.4 Diffraction at an isolated wall, $\theta_{crit} < \theta_w < 90°$; standard two- and three-shock theory for non-reactive media and the effects of reaction

Previous sections have shown that CCW theory results in a tolerable description of Mach reflection of detonation waves. However, the theory takes no account of the effects of liberation of chemical energy behind the incident wave, and it is difficult to incorporate appropriate modifications so to do. Although the fuel-lean mixtures, most likely to be produced by a malfunction of plant, minimize the effects of energy deposition and change in composition, it is appropriate to estimate their approximate magnitude. This is most readily accomplished in terms of standard two- and three-shock theory. While its application to non-reactive media is described in a number of texts (for instance, Liepman and Roshko [301]), a brief description is necessary in order to appreciate the required modifications to take chemical reactions into account.

Figure 6.11(a) shows, in stationary-shock coordinates, the flows associated with a regularly reflected shock. From a consideration of the continuity of mass, momentum and energy across incident (IO) and reflected (OR) shock, it can be shown that the angles of deflection, δ_1 and δ_2, are given by

$$\tan \delta_1 = \frac{(1 - \rho_1/\rho_2) \tan \omega_1}{\left[1 + \dfrac{\rho_1}{\rho_2} \tan^2 \omega_1\right]} \tag{6.12}$$

and

$$\tan \delta_2 = \frac{(1 - \rho_2/\rho_3) \tan (2\pi - \omega_2)}{\left[1 + \dfrac{\rho_2}{\rho_3} \tan^2 (2\pi - \omega_2)\right]} \tag{6.13}$$

Since the flow leaving the reflected shock must be parallel to the wedge $\delta_2 = -\delta_1$, and the effect of θ_w and M on the properties of the reflected wave can be computed using standard non-reactive shock theory, outlined in Chapter 2.

$$p_2/p_1 = \frac{2\gamma M^2 \sin^2 \omega_1 - (\gamma - 1)}{\gamma + 1} \tag{6.14}$$

$$\rho_2/\rho_1 = \frac{(\gamma + 1) M^2 \sin^2 \omega_1}{(\gamma - 1) M^2 \sin^2 \omega_1 + 2} \tag{6.15}$$

$$T_2/T_1 = \frac{[2M^2 \sin^2 \omega_1 - (\gamma - 1)][(\gamma - 1) M^2 \sin^2 \omega_1 + 2]}{(\gamma + 1) M^2 \sin^2 \omega_1} \tag{6.16}$$

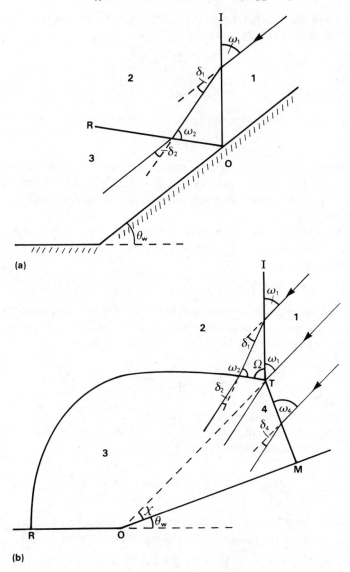

Figure 6.11 Flows into a regular reflection (a) and Mach reflection (b); IO and TI
incident wave, OR and TR reflected wave, TM Mach stem.

These equations result in two possible configurations for the reflected
wave. Experimental studies indicate that, in practice, the weaker front
results. For small values of θ_w the solution fails, predicting subsonic flow into
the reflected front. As we have seen, in this case, Mach reflection occurs. This

is shown in Fig. 6.11(b), again in stationary shock coordinates. The angles of incidence of flow now become

$$\omega_1 = 90° - (\theta_w + \chi) \tag{6.17}$$

and

$$\omega_4 = 90° - \chi \tag{6.18}$$

and the angle of deflection through the Mach stem

$$\delta_4 = \delta_1 + \delta_2 \tag{6.19}$$

With the component of Mach number normal to the Mach stem $M \sin \omega_4 / \sin \omega_1$, and for the pressures to be equal on either side of the slip stream ($p_3 = p_4$), the resultant equations can be solved to obtain the trajectory of the triple point, χ.

In order to take into account the energy released behind a detonation front [310], the equation for continuity of energy must be modified resulting in the combined equation

$$(\gamma + 1)M^2\rho_{12}^2 - 2(\gamma M^2 + 1)\rho_{12} + (\gamma - 1)M^2 + 2(1 + q) = 0 \tag{6.20}$$

where q is the ratio of chemical energy liberated to the initial energy of the gas and ρ_{12} the reciprocal of the density ratio across the front. If q is set equal to the heat released behind a C–J front, given by the standard relationship

$$q_{CJ} = \frac{(M_{CJ}^2 - 1)^2}{2(\gamma + 1)M_{CJ}^2} \tag{6.21}$$

then Equation 6.20 has only one solution.

Taking into account both $q \neq 0$ and a change in γ behind the front, the equation for the continuity of energy becomes

$$D_{CJ}^2 + \frac{2\gamma_1}{\gamma_1 - 1}\frac{p_1}{\rho_1}(1 + q) = u_2^2 + \frac{2\gamma_2}{\gamma_2 - 1}\frac{p_2}{\rho_2} \tag{6.22}$$

where u is the flow velocity and subscripts 1 and 2 refer to gas ahead and behind the front respectively. The analogous equation to (6.20) is

$$(\alpha_2 - 1)\gamma_1 M^2\rho_{12}^2 + \alpha_2(\gamma_1 M^2 + 1)\rho_{12} + \gamma_1 M^2 + \alpha_1(1 + q) = 0 \tag{6.23}$$

where $\alpha = 2\gamma/(\gamma - 1)$, and the equation corresponding to (6.19) is

$$q_{CJ} = \frac{(\alpha_2 - 2)^2\gamma_1 M_{CJ}^4 + 2\alpha_1^2\gamma_1 M_{CJ}^2 + \alpha_1^2 - 1}{4(\alpha_2 - 1)\alpha_1\gamma_1 M_{CJ}^2} \tag{6.24}$$

Using the standard relationship between shock strength and the reciprocal of the density ratio across the front

$$p_{21} = \gamma_1 M^2(1 - \rho_{12}) + 1 \tag{6.25}$$

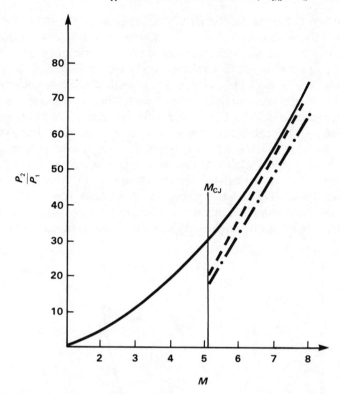

Figure 6.12   Theoretical influence of the Mach number of a detonation on its strength in $2H_2 + O_2 + Ar$ mixture, $M_{CJ} = 5.1$, $\gamma = 1.45$ [310]. ——— $q = 0$, $\gamma_1 = \gamma_2$; ·—·—· $q = q_{CJ}$, $\gamma_1 = \gamma_2$; —————$q = q_{CJ}$, $\gamma_1 = 1.45$, $\gamma_2 = 1.20$.

The combination of Equations 6.23 and 6.24 or 6.20 and 6.21 give the dependence of p_{21} on the Mach number of the front. Figure 6.12 shows results for a mixture of $2H_2 + O_2 + Ar$, $M_{CJ} = 5.10$, $\gamma_1 = 1.47$ and $\gamma_2 = 1.20$ [33]. Clearly, the effect of the addition of energy behind the incident front is to lessen its strength; however, the overall decrease in strength is reduced when the reduction in specific heat ratio is taken into account. As noted previously, the reduction in strength of the incident front from the commonly-used value, $q = 0$, will be less significant for the fuel-lean mixtures more likely to be encountered in practice. Furthermore, it is unlikely that accurate data on γ_2 will be available for such mixtures. For these reasons and because calculations with $q = 0$ result, in general, in overestimates of local pressures and therefore conservative design practices, their use is likely to continue.

It is possible to make some estimates of the effects of $q > 0$ and $\gamma \neq$ constant on local pressures produced by diffracting detonations. In order to do so, it is necessary to make some simplifying assumptions about the state of the gas behind the various shocks. One possibility for regular reflection is to calculate the deflection in flow behind the incident wave from the ratio of the velocity of gas at the C–J plane to the C–J velocity, using the standard zero deflection condition from two-shock theory. In order to specify q and γ_2 the flow behind the incident wave is assumed to be in thermal equilibrium. Similarly for Mach reflection, the gas behind the Mach stem can be assumed to be in thermal equilibrium at the enhanced temperature and pressure existing there. However, for $M_w \leq 1.3\, M_{CJ}$ there are negligible changes from γ_2 appropriate to an M_{CJ} wave. Figures 6.13 and 6.14 show a comparison of the effect of θ_w on the peak pressure ratio calculated from CCW theory (1), standard two- and three-shock theory (2) and the theory for $q \neq 0$ and $\gamma_1 \neq \gamma_2$ (3) for an argon-diluted stoichiometric mixture of hydrogen and oxygen and an undiluted stoichiometric mixture of acetylene and oxygen respectively [33]. For

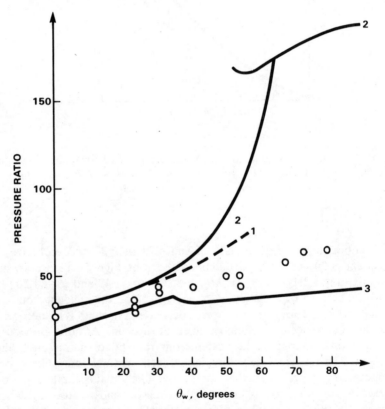

Figure 6.13 Influence of θ_w on the reduction in peak pressure ratio due to energy addition and change in γ [33]. $\bigcirc$, experimental results for $2H_2 + O_2 + Ar$, $M_{CJ} = 5.1$, $\gamma_1 = 1.45$ and $\gamma_2 = 1.20$; (1) CCW theory; (2) two- and three-shock theory; (3) reactive shock theory.

$\theta_w < 40°$ the non-reactive theories result in closely comparable predictions, but there is a pronounced decrease in the peak pressures predicted by reactive theory for all values of θ_w. Also shown on the plots are experimental results for the peak pressures generated in both mixtures. Since the measurements impose stringent requirements on the temporal resolution of pressure transducers, there must be some doubt as to the absolute accuracy of the measurements. However, this cannot fully account for the fact that reactive theory appears to perform well for the argon-diluted oxyhydrogen mixture, but not for the oxyacetylene mixture. Possibly the reactive theory performs better for mixtures with widely-spaced transverse fronts. Evidently the anomaly merits further experimental investigation, in the absence of which it appears that CCW theory is adequate for the purposes of design for $\theta_w < \theta_{crit}$, and that the more cumbersome reactive theory need only be applied at larger values of θ_w.

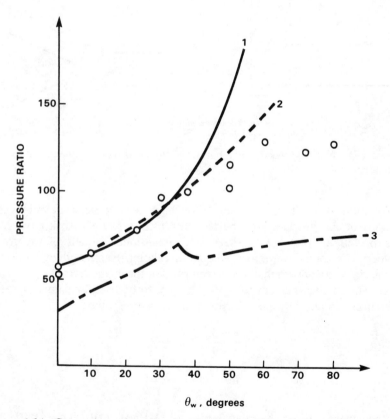

Figure 6.14 Comparison of predicted and measured peak pressure ratios on wedges of various angles. (1) CCW theory; (2) two- and three-shock theory; (3) reactive shock theory; $\bigcirc$ experimental results for $2C_2H_2 + 5O_2$, $M_{CJ} = 7.0$, $\gamma_1 = 1.36$ and $\gamma_2 = 1.20$, $S = 3$ mm.

6.5 Normal reflection of a detonation wave

Head-on reflection of part or all of a detonation can occur in a variety of configurations of plant. For example, a portion of the front, defined by the angle the head of the expansion makes with the original direction of the wall, may collide orthogonally with a portion of a sharp 90° bend or with the apex of a junction (Fig. 6.15). Again, following central initiation in a spherical vessel, the complete periphery will undergo normal reflection at the wall. There are, however, grave difficulties in defining the magnitude and durations of the pressures resulting from the reflection of real, as opposed to idealized,

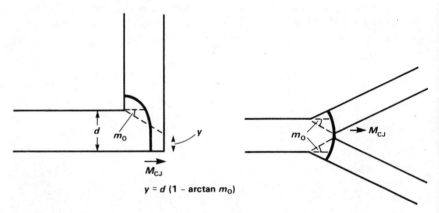

$$y = d\,(1 - \arctan m_0)$$

Figure 6.15   Normal reflection of a portion of (a) a C–J wave in a bend and (b) in a junction.

detonation waves. This may account for the paucity of experimental investigations of the process, and the fact that results of such work have been interpreted in terms of idealized one-dimensional models of the front. Indeed, it is not unknown for the equation relating the strength of a reflected shock $p_{52} = p_5/p_2$ with that of the reciprocal of the incident front $p_{12} = p_1/p_2$ in a non-reactive medium ($q = 0$, $\gamma_1 = \gamma_2$), to be used in estimating peak pressures produced by the reflection of a detonation wave

$$p_{52} = \frac{\left(\dfrac{\gamma+1}{\gamma-1}\right) + 2 - p_{12}}{1 + p_{12}\left(\dfrac{\gamma+1}{\gamma-1}\right)} \tag{6.26}$$

With values of p_{12} in the range typical of C–J waves ($0.1 > p_{12} > 0.02$) and values of γ typical of the unreacted medium, $\gamma = 1.3$, Equation 6.26 results in values of $p_{52} \leq 5$. From the previous discussion of the experimental results for pressure ratios across the reflected wave in stoichiometric mixtures of oxyacetylene and oxyhydrogen, when it was shown that $p_{52} \leq 2.5$, Equation 6.26 evidently produces excessive overestimates of peak pressures.

An outline of some of the problems in treating the head-on reflection of a multi-dimensional detonation should assist in indicating the reasons why oversimplified analyses are frequently employed. In addition, it serves to identify the mechanisms whereby wide variations in local pressures occur and the difficulties in specifying the locations at which they are produced. Figure 6.16 shows an incident detonation ITX, with widely spaced transverse waves

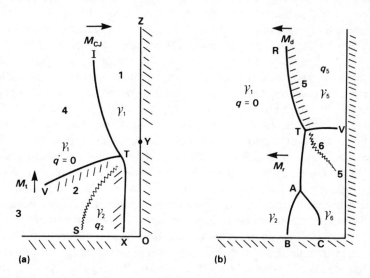

Figure 6.16   Local variations in conditions during the normal reflection of a structured detonation. ITX, incident detonation; TV, transverse wave; TS, slipstream; OY, portion of wall experiencing detonation reflection; YZ, portion of wall experiencing shock reflection; RT, detonation front; TA, reflected shock, BAC, bifurcated reflected shock; //////, reaction zones.

of average velocity M_t, approaching a wall at an average velocity of M_{CJ}. In region 1, between the front and the walls, the properties of the medium are those of the original mixture. Region 2 contains the products of reaction zones behind the Mach stem and transverse front. The composition of these can be estimated from the assumption that they are in thermal equilibrium in a flow initially treated by a Mach stem of velocity 1.3 M_{CJ}, so that the strength of the reflected shock from the diffraction of the planar portion of TX can be calculated from Equations 6.23–6.25. Well behind the reaction zones, say at about 5 S, is region 3, with the main expansion fan resulting in the curvature of the natural transverse front. The mixture in the flow in region 4 is compressed along the periphery to pressures ranging from that appropriate to a wave of velocity of M_{CJ} to that appropriate to a wave of 0.6 M_{CJ}. However, it has not reacted so that $\gamma = \gamma_1$ and $q = 0$. Close to the reflecting face the strength of the reflected shock is given by Equation 6.26, using appropriate local values for the incident front. The increase in temperature and pressure behind this reflected shock front will result in a reaction zone forming close behind it, and a transition to a reflected detonation, TR, as shown. While the highest local pressures are likely to be generated behind the reflected detonation in region 5 close to TV, there is no obvious way in which to calculate them. Note that Equation 6.26 is derived on the basis of stagnant mixture behind a non-reactive shock and that $\gamma_5 \neq \gamma_2$ and $q_5 \neq q_2$. Additional problems arise in estimating local pressures further from the end face, when detonations are confined in tubes or channels. These problems result from the bifurcation of the reflected wave as it propagates back through the thickening boundary layer, left by the incident front. The process of bifurcation is promoted in gases of low γ, so is of particular importance in the products of a detonation.

There are a number of alternative treatments of the normal reflection of a detonation, all based on highly idealized fronts and generally using the ZND model [311–315]. As such they result in some average pressure, well below the local peaks to be expected from the reflection of a structured front. Thus, early models took into account the effects of changes in γ behind the incident front, but not directly the influence of energy addition. A somewhat more general treatment accounting for the effects of a change in γ and those of the Taylor expansion wave behind a planar reaction front has been suggested [316]; however, there must be some doubt as to the accuracy of its predictions, even for the most ideal fronts which can be obtained experimentally. For instance, although the theory predicts the expected acceleration of the reflected shock as it travels back through the Taylor expansion, it over-estimates the final steady velocity, giving 2.2 mm μs^{-1}, compared with the experimental value of 1.9 mm μs^{-1}. The experimental result was obtained in a stoichiometric oxyhydrogen mixture at an initial pressure of 10 bar, in order to minimize departures from unidimensionality.

In addition to the difficulties imposed in locating the regions of peak pressure, in the absence of a knowledge of the positions of the transverse waves at the instant of reflection, analogous difficulties arise in predicting the shape of the pressure histories. The durations of the peak pressures are given very approximately by nS/v_r, where nS is the distance between the leading portion of the front and the C–J plane and v_r the velocity of the reflected shock, which can vary across the front on account of changes in the medium into which it propagates, and along the length of confinement due to bifurcation. In marginally-detonable media nS may be as large as 100 mm, and with mean velocities of reflected shock of ≤ 2 mm μs^{-1}, the durations of peak pressures may be up to tens of microseconds. For more readily-detonable media, where nS is much shorter, durations can be as low as microseconds or fractions thereof – indeed, experimental measurements of the durations of peak pressures in stoichiometric mixtures of oxygen and hydrogen, using pressure transducers of very short rise-times, suggest that times at half-peak height are less than a microsecond [309].

6.6 Transmission of a planar detonation through an abrupt expansion in area

The propagation of an initially planar detonation through a sudden change in area has received much more attention than have interactions with any other forms of confinement [35, 89, 99, 118, 124]. There are a number of reasons for this, some of which were hinted at in Chapter 5. Most importantly from a practical point of view, it is necessary to be able to account fully for the effects of the properties of the medium on the critical diameter of the inlet for the establishment of a steady hemispherical detonation (d_c), in order to secure a sound foundation for the design of devices for quenching detonations. The problems associated with producing an analysis of the mechanisms governing the transition from steady and planar to steady and curved fronts are mitigated slightly in an abrupt change by the fact that symmetry about the axis is preserved throughout the process. Consequently, there is an attractive prospect of relating the critical diameter to the critical energy, E_c, for the initiation of a spherical detonation. Making use of the information on diffraction at a wall $\theta_w < 0°$ (Section 6.2), we now examine in some depth the progress which has been made in developing a general theory.

Consider for simplicity a planar shock in a non-reactive medium travelling through a nozzle of diameter d_o into a tank with $\theta_w = 90°$. Figure 6.17 shows the shock envelope within the tank prior to the heads of the expansion fan converging on the axis of symmetry [294]. A truncated cone, with its front edge continuing to propagate at the Mach number of the incident front, exists within the decaying shock envelope. The angle of the cone is defined by the vector sum of sound speed and gas velocity within it (Equation 6.1). A similar situation pertains to a planar detonation with a pressure p and gas velocity u in the truncated cone, appropriate to a front of C–J velocity D_{CJ}, doing work on the mixture at lower pressure in the surrounding envelope. Arguably, the simplest possible relationship between critical energies and diameters is obtained by equating twice the work done, w (to account for spherical symmetry), with the critical energy [258]; thus

$$w \sim \int_0^{t_c} p u_{CJ} A \, dt \tag{6.27}$$

where A is the area of the truncation, u_{CJ} is the gas velocity behind a C–J front and t_c is the time at which the heads of the expansion fan cross at the axis of symmetry. Then,

$$t_c = \frac{L}{S}\left(\frac{r_c - r_o}{D_{CJ}}\right) \tag{6.28}$$

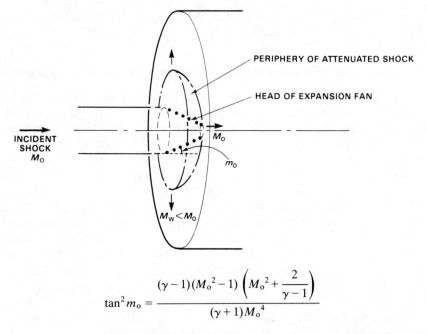

$$\tan^2 m_o = \frac{(\gamma - 1)(M_o{}^2 - 1)\left(M_o{}^2 + \dfrac{2}{\gamma - 1}\right)}{(\gamma + 1)M_o{}^4}$$

Figure 6.17   The attenuation of shock in a sudden expansion in area [294, 295]

where L and S are the length and width of a detonation cell respectively. Integrating Equation 6.28 and expressing the results in terms of d_c and d_o on the assumption that $E_c = 2w$ gives

$$E_c = \left(\frac{\pi p_{CJ} u_{CJ}}{4 D_{CJ}}\right)\frac{L}{S}\left(\frac{d_c}{d_o} - 1\right)^3 \qquad (6.29)$$

Figure 6.18 shows values of E_c calculated from Equation 6.29, using the measured values of d_c listed in Table 5.3 for a number of hydrocarbons in stoichiometric mixtures with oxygen and air. The theory, shown by the line, consistently underestimates the experimental results (open circles), but clearly predicts the correct trend of a steep increase in E_c with increasing values of d_c. Some caution is advisable in extending the use of Equation 6.29 to fuels other than hydrocarbons and oxidants other than oxygen, especially in media in which detonations produce large sizes of cells. Then, the analogy between non-reactive shocks and detonations breaks down, since the flow behind the unattenuated portion of the front is no longer parallel with the axis of symmetry; there must be doubts as to the applicability of the standard relationship $L = 0.6S$ to such media.

Another approach to the problem of estimating critical diameters, which

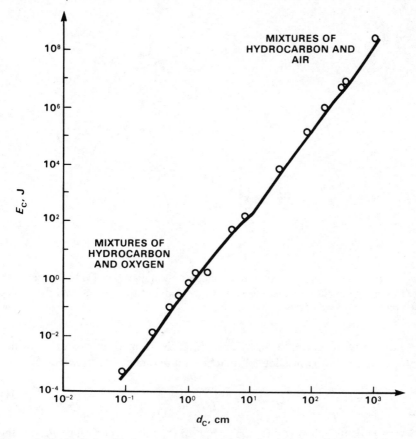

Figure 6.18 Relationship between critical energies for mixtures of hydrocarbon and oxidant and critical diameter; line taken from 'work-done' concept [258] and ○, experimental results [259].

has been applied to liquid explosives [317] but should be equally appropriate to gaseous mixtures is illustrated in Fig. 6.19. Here the paths of the triple points behind the unattenuated portion of the front are shown as full lines, the reaction zones by the hatched lines and the trajectory of the head of the expansion by a dotted line. Considering the flow field in a frame of reference fixed at the boundary of the unattenuated front, A, molecules entering at A will react, provided that they are not cooled in the expansion wave BB′ before their residence time t_s exceeds the chemical induction period t_c in region 3. The velocity of BB′ relative to A is $(u_3 - a_3)$, where u and a are particle and sonic velocities in region 3, so that

$$(u_3 - a_3)t_c = u_3 t_s \qquad (6.30)$$

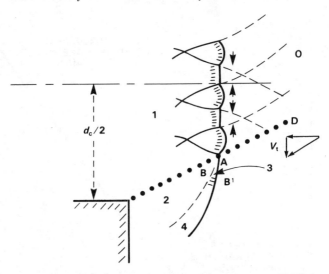

Figure 6.19 Dremin and Trofimov model for critical diameters [317]; hatched lines representing reaction zones, dashed lines trajectories of triple points and dotted line the path of the head of the expansion fan.

Following reaction, a transverse front is formed in region 3 which propagates in both directions. It reaches A after an interval t_A, given by

$$t_A = \frac{u_3 t_s}{D_3 - u_3} \tag{6.31}$$

where D_3 is its velocity in region 3. For an inlet of the critical diameter, the transverse wave must arrive at the axis of symmetry in a time $(t_A + t_c)$ where

$$t_A + t_c = \frac{d_c}{2v_t} \tag{6.32}$$

and v_t is the velocity of the transverse wave. Combining the equations results in

$$d_c = 2u_3 v_t t_s \left[\frac{1}{(D_3 - u_3)} + \frac{1}{(u_3 - a_3)} \right] \tag{6.33}$$

Experimental measurements of v_t suggest that it is close to a_3. With v_t equated to a_3, Equation 6.33 has been shown to predict d_c for liquid TNT and nitromethane.

The attractive feature of the analysis is the direct use of the chemical induction time, although it contains a number of features of somewhat doubtful generality. The most obvious of these is the assumption that uniform conditions exist in region 3. When values appropriate to a C–J front in a stoichiometric mixture of oxygen and acetylene are substituted into Equation 6.33, the predicted value of d_c is between one and two orders of magnitude too small.

A more elegant approach is possible [35]. This involves combining the Shchelkin instability criterion [318] (to take account of the chemical processes) with CCW theory (to deal with fluid dynamic aspects). Whilst it extends both of these to their limits of applicability and is rather complex, it provides a clearer understanding of the mechanisms involved in the transition from a planar to a hemispherical detonation. The Shchelkin criterion suggests that a detonation fails when an increase in induction time, Δt_c, occurs such that the ratio $\Delta t_c/t_c \geq 1$. With the steady-state induction period related to the density ρ_{CJ} and temperature T_{CJ} behind a shock of C–J velocity in standard Arrhenius form:

$$t_c = \frac{A}{\rho_{CJ}}\exp(E/RT_{CJ}) \qquad (6.34)$$

where A is a constant related to collision frequency and E a global activation energy.

Substituting the standard Rankine–Hugoniot relationship results in the Shchelkin criterion becoming $\Delta M_{CJ}/M_{CJ} \sim 0.1$ for typical values of E and M_{CJ}. In other words, a planar detonation is quenched when the velocity of the leading front falls to $0.9\,M_{CJ}$, in fair agreement with experimental studies which suggest failure occurs at about $0.8\,M_{CJ}$, so that $0.1\,M_{CJ} \leq \Delta M_{CJ} \leq 0.2\,M_{CJ}$.

Taking the Shchelkin criterion as $\partial M_o/\partial y = \Delta M_{CJ}/L$ and referring to Fig. 6.20, a sketch of the coordinate system for a CCW treatment, the problem is

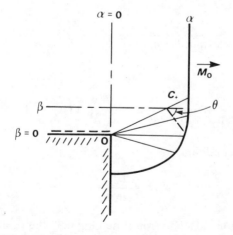

Figure 6.20 CCW coordinate system for diffraction of a detonation in a sudden change in area.

to define $\partial M_o / \partial y$, where y is the distance travelled by the diffracted wall shock. The position of the precursor front is defined by $\alpha = a_o t = $ constant, where a_o is the speed of sound in the undisturbed medium. Again, the particle paths close to the leading front are defined by $\beta = $ constant. Centred at the inlet of the expansion, the Prandtl–Meyer fan results in the C_+ characteristics being straight lines. The Mach number and the inclination of the particle paths with respect to the x-coordinate, $\theta(M)$, are also constant along each C_+ characteristic with $\theta(M)$ given by

$$\theta(M) = n^{0.5}(\cosh^{-1} M - \cosh^{-1} M_o) \qquad (6.35)$$

where n has the values defined in Table 6.1 for media of different γ. The angle between the leading C_+ characteristic and a particle path behind the unattenuated front, m_o, has been defined by Equation 6.2 and gives the relationship between the coordinates of the particle paths, α and β, and the leading shock, x and y. Integrating Equation 6.35 along a C_+ characteristic results in

$$x_s = \frac{\alpha M_o \cos(\theta + m_o)}{\cos m_o} \quad \text{and} \quad y_s = \frac{\alpha M_o \sin(\theta + m_o)}{\cos m_o} \qquad (6.36)$$

Since we require the value of $\partial M_o / \partial y$ near the head of the expansion fan and $M_o = M_{CJ} \gg 1$, Equation 6.36 simplifies to

$$\left(\frac{\partial M_o}{\partial y}\right) x_s = \frac{M_{CJ}}{x_s[\tan(\theta + m_o) + n^{0.5}]} \qquad (6.37)$$

so that

$$\frac{M_{CJ}}{x_s[\tan(\theta + m_o) + n^{0.5}]} = \frac{\Delta M_{CJ}}{L} \qquad (6.38)$$

or

$$\frac{1}{[\tan(\theta + m_o) + n^{0.5}]} = \left(\frac{x_s}{2S}\right)\left(\frac{\Delta M_{CJ}}{M_{CJ}}\right) \qquad (6.39)$$

and for the critical condition

$$x_s = \frac{d_c}{2 \tan m_o} \qquad (6.40)$$

Thus, it is possible to calculate from Equation 6.39 the position at which a hemispherical wave should be established, and from a combination of Equations 6.39 and 6.40 the critical diameter. In both cases the predicted

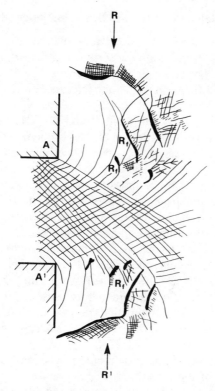

Figure 6.21 Sketch of a soot track record of the re-establishment of a detonation in $2C_2H_2 + 5O_2$, S = 1.3 mm in an abrupt expansion: AA′ = inlet; RR′ = predicted re-establishment plane and R_f = failed attempts at re-initiation [35].

results are generally within a factor of 2 of experimental measurements, on mixtures which produce a well-defined and fine structure of transverse fronts.

An idealized sketch of a soot track record, Fig. 6.21 illustrates the re-establishment of a detonation in a stoichiometric mixture of acetylene and oxygen propagating through a suddenly expanding channel [35]. Regions of high pressure, associated with patches of fine writing, result from failing attempts at reinitiation, R_f. The arrows at RR′ mark the positions, predicted from Equation 6.39, at which a steady curved detonation should be produced. In this instance the prediction underestimates the transition distance, but corresponds reasonably closely with the start of attempts at reinitiation. Further work is needed before firm recommendations can be made on the choice of the most appropriate treatment of diffraction in abrupt expansions; however, the combined CCW–Shchelkin criterion treatment does serve to identify positions at which anomalously high pressures are to be expected, following attempts at re-establishment.

6.7 Propagation of detonations through bends and junctions

In view of the facts that the most common form of detonation is one occurring in a channel or pipeline and that typical runs of pipework in chemical plant contain a number of bends and junctions, surprisingly little work has been carried out on the diffraction of detonations in different forms of these components. There have however been a number of studies of shocks in non-reactive media propagating through bends [319–321] and junctions [322, 323]. In general, these confirm that the profiles of the front at expansive and compressive surfaces are reasonably accurately estimated in the early stages of the process by CCW theory. These simplified analyses only fail when the resultant wave systems set up at opposing walls start to interact. Thus, it is possible to estimate the peak local pressure, resulting from the normal reflection of a portion of the predicted profile, the strength of which has been defined by the methods outlined. An important feature to note is that good design practice can reduce the departure of the experimental profile from the predicted, and thus reduce the possibility of the occurrence of unexpectedly high local pressures. This can be achieved by ensuring that any change in confinement is designed to be as gradual as possible. It allows sufficient distance for the completion of interactions between the various wave systems and so ensures that departures from their averaged properties, given by the predictive technique, are minimized [324].

Similar considerations apply to detonations in bends and junctions. An experimental study of the effect of radius curvature R of a $90°$ bend in a channel, half-height r, on the shape of shocks and detonations propagating through it, suggested that the reduction in asymmetry observed to occur with non-reactive shocks in channels with $R/r \geq 5$ was mirrored by the behaviour of detonations [296, 325]. However, there are indications that the later stages of the interactions of a detonation, especially one with widely-spaced transverse fronts, with a bend are much more complex than those of a non-reactive shock. For instance, although steady detonations were observed to be re-established in, or downstream of, all the bends tested, both the distances required for stabilization and the positions at which higher than C–J pressures were generated depended on the configuration of the bend. Figure 6.22 is a smoked foil record of a detonation with widely-spaced transverse waves in a sharp $90°$ bend. A steady front is eventually formed some diameters downstream of the bend, following the reflection of the wall-generated triple point $0_1 0_2 0_3$ at the inner wall. Note particularly, the patch of fine writing, representing a region of high pressure, just downstream of 0_3. Although in this instance there are similar but much less extensive regions close to the compressive surface, the largest regime of high pressure occurs (somewhat surprisingly at first sight) on the expansive surface. Since the processes involved are intrinsic to detonations, in the investigation of an explosion, damage to the inner wall of a bend may serve to discriminate between deflagrations and detonations.

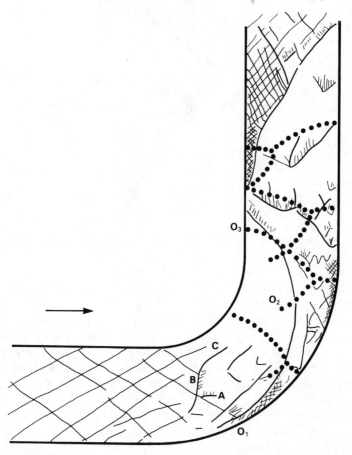

Figure 6.22 Sketch of a smoked foil record of re-establishment of a detonation in a sharp bend, following reflection of triple point, trajectory $O_1O_2O_3$ at inner wall [325], • • • shock profiles in a non-reactive medium.

6.8 Interaction of a detonation with an inert surrounding gas

Although, as will become apparent, it is possible to suggest safety measures which involve surrounding an explosive medium with an inert and compressible gas [326, 327], Chapter 6 appears the appropriate place to deal with the subject. This is because the mechanisms governing the interaction are related to those described in previous sections. Early work indicated that it was possible to sustain detonations, propagating at stable velocities of as low as half the C–J value [116, 328], in detonable mixtures surrounded by an inert gas of lower density. However, questions about the possible effects of thin diaphragms [329], used to separate the media, and about the influence of diffusion across the boundary in the absence of a diaphragm, have resulted in some doubts as to whether such fronts are truly steady. Recently, the concept

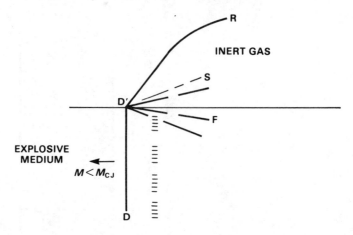

Figure 6.23 Detonation quenching by inert and compressible boundary layers [331].

of the apparent stability in velocity being a facet of the very slow process of quenching is gaining favour [330].

Figure 6.23 is a representation of the quenching of a unidimensional detonation front DD′, which occurs via the production of an oblique shock (D′R) in the inert gas and a resultant expansion fan (D′F) stretching back into the reaction zone. This causes the deceleration of the front to produce a deflagration, travelling at the velocity of sound in the inert gas. D′S is the contact surface separating gas treated by the oblique shock from that treated by the incident front. Based on such an idealized model [331], it has been suggested that detonations in channels of widths less than the length of the reaction zone should be quenched. Recalling the uncertainties in predictions of hydrodynamic thicknesses of detonation fronts and their likely wide variations with changing stoichiometry and nature of the fuel, however, there must be some doubt as to general utility of such a criterion in specifying pipeline bores or the appropriate characteristics of packings. Nevertheless, there is a case to be made for the consideration of basing the design of quenching devices for pipeline detonations on some form of inert and compressible medium. The major problem lies in ensuring the continued separation of the explosive and inert layers. One possible solution is a plastic foam liner containing an inert gas such as helium or, perhaps less effectively, nitrogen. In this context the ability of a rigid polyurethane foam to mitigate shock loading of structures is of interest [332].

6.9 Refraction of detonations in mixtures of different composition

A detonation propagating through a mixture of fuel and oxidant, created by the leakage of a high-pressure reservoir of either component, will encounter wide changes in composition. In such a case these changes are likely to be in the form of gradients existing over extended distances. In chemical processing plant it is also possible to conceive of circumstances in which a sharply defined change in composition occurs. There is a strong interest from the practical point of view in the effects of changes in speed of sound, in ratio of specific heats and in chemical energy available on the process of refraction, particularly on the distances over which the properties of the leading front adjust to accommodate these changes.

An early appreciation of the complexities of the processes came as a by-product of studies of the initiation of confined detonations, in which the source was a steady detonation front in a standard mixture [333]. The steady front ruptured a diaphragm separating the source and test medium, resulting in a stable detonation, or the decay of the initiating front to a uniform velocity in the test medium, in some cases as far as 50 diameters downstream of the diaphragm. In the absence of a diaphragm, the distance required for the formation of a stable front in the test mixture was reduced by a factor of about ten.

There appears to have been only one detailed study of the refraction of a detonation at an interface between two different, gaseous, explosive mixtures, separated by a thin diaphragm [334]. This involved the investigation of spinning fronts in a mixture of methane and oxygen refracting in an oxymethane mixture of different stoichiometry, with a systematic examination of the effects of varying the angle of incidence. Similar studies in inert media [335] are explicable in terms of Paterson's [336] classical analysis, latterly extended to detonation fronts [337] which describes the properties of the transmitted shock and those of the shock or rarefaction fan reflected back across the interface, depending on the match of acoustic impedance there. The experiments with detonations revealed some of the additional complexities, brought about by the presence of reaction zones, which appeared to be enhanced when the front travelled from a medium of high C–J velocity into one of lower velocity. Similar effects on the transverse fronts have been noted, with a slow decay on detonations propagating across a fast–slow interface. However, it is not possible from these experiments to draw any inference on rates at which stable velocities were regained.

There have been a number of studies of the transmission of detonations through shallow gradients in composition [338, 339]. However, the experimental techniques in some of these are open to criticism. The removal of a simple diaphragm in a horizontal tube is likely to produce sufficient mixing for the use of gradients calculated from diffusional theory to be inappropriate [338]. There does seem to be general agreement that the changes in velocity of the transmitted front closely mirror those in composition [307, 338, 339]. This is not surprising, when the analogy with a detonation travelling through a gradual change in area is made. Then, the averaging out of the effects of the various interacting wave systems is rapid. Consequently, it seems safe to assume that high local pressures, resulting from the slow decay of overdriven detonations, are unlikely to persist in gaseous media of changing composition over long distances.

6.10 Concluding remarks

It will have become apparent that systematic studies have only recently been made of the interactions of detonations with changes in confinement, typical of those encountered in chemical plant. The initial objectives of such work were generally to define the peaks in pressure produced by diffraction and, if possible, to pinpoint the area in which they occur in order to specify the design of plant which could safely contain such loads. A potentially valuable by-product of a successful outcome of such investigations would have been the identification of features distinguishing the local pressure profiles produced by detonations from those resulting from deflagrations.

The briefest summary of experimental work done to date is to suggest that it emphasizes the dangers associated with an oversimplified approach to the design of plant which may be subjected to the effects of a detonation. For instance, although it is possible to estimate approximately the factors by which pressures, predicted by simple unidimensional theories for certain changes in shape, are enhanced, the accuracy of such estimates decreases as the composition of media approaches its limits of detonability. Furthermore, the apparently simplest case to analyse for such mixtures, that of normal reflection of a detonation at a closed end of a tube, is in fact possibly the most complex of all. Indeed, there is at present no reliable method for dealing with the dual effects of the reflection of a leading shock which results in the formation of a reflected detonation and of its rapid bifurcation. Finally, unless great care is taken in designing any changes in cross-section to be gradual, there is little prospect of safe containment being based solely on the strengthening of an isolated portion of the change in shape. This is not to dismiss the case for further experiments on the interaction of non-planar detonation waves, typical of marginal media, with different shapes of components. In addition to increasing our understanding of the basic mechanisms involved, further experiments could well identify further phenomena distinguishing between detonations and deflagrations.

7

Damage caused by detonations

7.1 Introduction

The recent book by Baker *et al.* [340] covers in considerable detail the response of structures to the loads imposed by a blast front and contains valuable information on the resultant damage to buildings, to various forms of containment and to vehicles, and discusses the possibilities of injury to personnel. These features are described principally in terms of the freely-expanding spherical front produced by the detonation of a charge of condensed explosive or the rupture of an approximately spherical vessel filled with gas at high pressure. As such, the information is directly applicable to the blast front formed in the atmosphere surrounding, for instance, a detonating cloud, resulting from a fuel–air explosive weapon [341].

The existence of such a readily available source of information on the effects of the N-shaped pressure histories, with well defined variations in the durations of positive and negative phases characteristic of blast fronts, precludes the need for further discussion here. Furthermore, because of the wide variations in amplitudes and durations of the pressure profiles engendered by detonations in marginally-detonable gaseous mixtures, we have not included studies of damage in which attempts have been made to model the effects of gaseous detonations by charges of condensed explosives. These considerations result in severe limitations to data directly applicable to damage produced by detonations in fuel-lean mixtures. Thus, experimental studies have been carried out in stoichiometric mixtures and incidents in plant have been associated with mixtures of unknown composition.

We have chosen to dismiss the possibility of significant thermal damage resulting from a detonation. This is a reasonable assumption, on account of the high C–J velocities associated with a steady front and the relatively slow processes of heat transfer by conduction and convection; however, there may be special cases in which it *is* necessary to consider thermal effects. For instance, the walls containing detonable media may be flammable – burning of PVC and Perspex walls of detonation tubes in the flow of oxidizing products behind the leading shock front has been observed [342]. Again, it may be necessary to examine radiation from the flow behind a front in a suspension of dust in an oxidizing gas, in an analogous fashion to Moore and Weinberg's analysis [255] of radiation from large clouds of gases. The role of long path length in increasing emissivity in such clouds may be replaced by the increased density of the suspension brought about by shock compression.

Of closer relevance to more general cases of damage caused by detonation waves are studies of the effects of shock fronts in non-reactive gases on structures within or on the walls of conventional shock tubes. In these the high-pressure gas is separated from the low pressure test gas by a diaphragm. When this ruptures, the high-pressure gas acts as a piston, driving a series of pressure waves into the test gas. Since these waves have the property of heating the gas and consequently increasing the speed of sound therein, successive pulses coalesce to form a shock front some distance downstream of the diaphragm. By varying the pressure ratio across the diaphragm and choosing a high-pressure gas such as hydrogen or helium, the resultant shock can be of Mach number up to four, travelling supersonically relative to the cold gas ahead of it but subsonically in relation to the hot flow behind it. Whilst the Mach numbers of shocks in conventional shock tubes, and consequently pressure ratios across them, are generally below C–J values, it is possible to approach C–J levels in specially designed tubes. In addition, by a suitable choice of lengths of high pressure and test sections, it is possible to model the Taylor expansion front of a detonation by the expansion fan reflected from the high-pressure end of a conventional shock tube. The non-steady interactions of such shocks with changes in the shape of confinement have recently been exhaustively reviewed, so that information on how local pressures vary with time is readily available [297].

A number of studies of non-reactive shocks, albeit carried out without attempting to simulate the load histories imposed by detonations, have revealed a number of features which are likely to be equally relevant to detonations and are worthy of mention. The experimental studies of the strains produced in the aluminium walls of a shock tube by both incident and reflected waves [343] were found to be adequately described by thin-shell theory [344]. In addition, the strain profiles in the inelastic regime suggested that a zone of relaxation of strain occurred a millisecond or so behind the front. Similar experiments demonstrated that walls of polycarbonate and Perspex behaved very differently, with polycarbonate walls apparently being subjected to some plastic deformation before fragmenting into two or three pieces [345]. However, Perspex behaved in a brittle fashion, shattering into some thousands of fragments with a wide range of size distribution. The results led to the proposed use of such a test to complement or to replace the Charpy impact test.

A number of approaches can be used to demonstrate that the maximum force exerted on a plate by a suddenly applied load F_m, of much longer duration than the time constant of the surface can be up to twice that produced by a slowly-applied load of the same amplitude. Following Cole [346], and considering dynamic stressing in terms of the response of a spring, stiffness k to a mass m at the opposite end to its fixing, then the restoring force F on the mass displaced a distance x is given by

$$F = kx \tag{7.1}$$

For a force of P the equation of motion is

$$m\frac{d^2x}{dt^2} + kx = P \tag{7.2}$$

where $P = 0$ when $0 > t > t_1$ and $P = P_0$ when $0 < t < t_1$. Equation 7.2 has the

$$F = kx = A \cos \omega t + B \sin \omega t + P \tag{7.3}$$

solution where $\omega = \sqrt{(k/m)}$ and A and B are constants of integration. With boundary conditions $x = dx/dt = 0$ at $t = 0$, and x and dx/dt being continuous, then

$$F = P(1 - \cos \omega t), 0 < t < t_1 \tag{7.4}$$

and

$$F = P[\sin \omega t_1 \sin \omega t - (1 - \cos \omega t_1) \cos \omega t], t_1 < t \tag{7.5}$$

The maximum force at $t_1 = \pi/\omega$ is $2P$ and the deflection produced by a step pulse of long duration can be up to twice that produced by a slowly applied load.

The deformation of thin plates of various metals at the end of the test section of a conventional shock tube, subjected to appropriately lengthy pressure pulses behind the reflected fronts, has been studied [347]. In general, the observed ratio of deformation given by the rapidly-applied pulse to that given by a slowly-applied load was less than two, and depended on the degree of deformation and the properties of the plate, such as the degree of annealing. Arguably more importantly, when the plates were subjected to large deformations, they no longer behaved in ideal fashion, tending towards a conical shape for aluminium and mild steel and showing three or four separate protruberances for annealed copper. Figure 7.1 shows a comparison of the shapes of aluminium discs treated by a slowly-applied load and reflected shock wave, showing spherical distortion in the former case and the departures from sphericity at the centre (>25 mm) in the dynamically deformed disc.

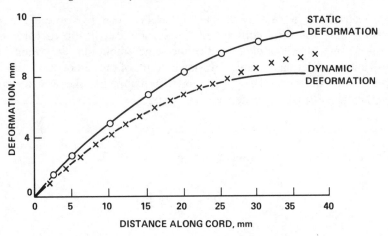

Figure 7.1 Conical deformation of aluminium discs subjected to the load imposed by the reflection of a non-reactive shock [347].

7.2 Early experiments on effective pressures generated by detonations

Early experiments measuring the properties of detonations [19, 162] were particularly elegant and served as a source of inspiration for a number of further studies [348, 349]. They included probably the only systematic study of the mutual reflection of detonation waves meeting head-on [349]. Following investigation of available devices for measurement of pressure, the painstaking technique of using glass tubes of steadily increasing thickness of wall to contain the loads imposed by detonations was chosen. Tubes of similar thickness were then calibrated by bursting them hydraulically. Unfortunately, there is some evidence for the anomalous behaviour of glass subjected to rapidly-applied loads. Thus, it has been observed that the probability of glass tubes being shattered by a detonation was reduced by cooling the walls, although (as might be expected) continued stressing by treatment with a number of detonations increased the probability of failure [288]. Additional difficulties seem to have arisen in the earlier studies of mutual reflection of detonation waves [348], with the junction in the tube dividing a single front to form the colliding waves and with the bends in these tubes bringing the conjuncture of the fronts, causing partial extinction of the colliding waves. Investigation indicated that the reflection brought about an insignificant increase in pressure. Later experiments [349], in which careful attention was paid to the construction of the junctions and the bends, demonstrated an increase in the pressure on the mutual reflection of detonations in a $C_2N_2 + 2O_2$ mixture from 58 to 75 bar. The measurement of effective pressure of the incident front lies approximately midway between the theoretical peak of about 88 bar, and the C–J level, about 44 bar. A somewhat higher increase in pressure than that observed might be expected on reflection; however, to interpret this in terms of the effective pressure would require much more information on the properties of the front and on the behaviour of the walls.

Recognizing the need for an improved technique of measurement of pressure, Campbell *et al.* [350] chose to use the peripheral shearing of copper discs from which detonation waves were reflected. The discs were calibrated by a slowly-applied pneumatic load, relying on the shearing properties

Table 7.1 Effective pressures generated behind reflected detonations in various mixtures [350].

Mixture	Thickness of sheared disc (mm)	Thickness of containing disc (mm)	Best estimate of effective pressure (bar)	Pressure calculated for an incident C–J wave [31] (bar)
$C_2H_4 + 2O_2$	0.94	1.19	41.5	38.6
$C_2H_4 + 3O_2$	0.79	0.94	34.0	33.5
$2C_2H_4 + 13O_2$	0.58	0.74	26.0	25.8
$C_2H_4 + 19O_2$	0.48	0.55	19.0	16.0
$CH_4 + O_2$	0.79	0.94	34.0	31.2
$CH_4 + 2O_2$	0.79	0.94	31.0	28.8
$CH_4 + 4O_2$	0.58	0.74	26.0	23.2
$CH_4 + 8O_2$	0.55	0.58	22.4	17.6
$C_2H_2 + O_2$	0.94	1.19	41.5	37.5
$2C_2H_2 + 5O_2$	0.79	0.94	34.0	33.0
$2C_2H_2 + 15O_2$	0.58	0.74	26.0	21.2
$C_2H_2 + 10O_2$	0.55	–	>21.8	19.3
$2H_2 + O_2$	0.48	0.55	20.4	18.6
$7H_2 + O_2$	0.38	0.48	15.0	15.0
$2H_2 + 6O_2$	0.38	0.48	15.0	14.1
$2CO + O_2$	0.55	0.58	23.0	

remaining similar for dynamic and slowly-applied loads. The effective pressure was taken as the minimum thickness of disc withstanding shear under the load imposed by the detonation. Table 7.1 shows a selection of Campbell's results for various fuels mixed with oxygen, for thickness of discs containing the reflection of the wave and shearing under the load together with their estimate of effective pressure. Also shown are the pressures calculated for a C–J wave in these mixtures. It will be recalled that these are approximately half the peak pressures behind the wave. Further enhancement in pressure occurs on reflection, so that the effective pressures are well below the actual values. Figure 7.2 shows a selection of the results plotted as effective pressures against the C–J pressure calculated from experimental measurements of the velocity of the front for mixtures in which it has been measured.

$$P_{CJ} \simeq \frac{\gamma M^2}{\gamma + 1} \tag{7.6}$$

It serves to illustrate again that the measured values are well below those which must occur on reflection. Furthermore, it suggests a possible change in mechanism of the failure at pressures of >20 bar behind the C–J wave, where the curve of effective pressure levels out for detonations of increasing Mach number. However, there is some ambiguity as to whether complete peripheral shearing was at all times the criterion for failure; certainly photographs of unholed specimens reveal almost conical extension of the discs. It is possible that circumferential failure at the highest pressures was connected with sufficient acceleration of the centre of the disc for the disc to thin preferentially around the clamping device.

Scattered throughout earlier literature, there are a number of further descriptions of damage caused by detonations. For instance, Payman and Shepherd [351] refer to the opening of slits 1.5 m in length in an explosion gallery filled with a stoichiometric mixture of methane and air which detonated. In general, however, too little information is available on the

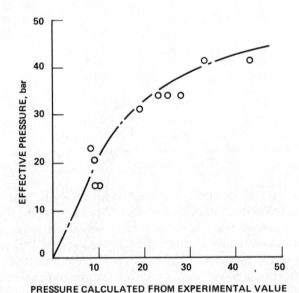

Figure 7.2 Comparison of pressures measured on the reflection of a detonation with C–J pressures [350].

position of initiation, changes in the shape of confinement, the mechanical properties of the containment and the uniformity of composition of the mixture, to draw any conclusions on effective pressures.

7.3 Damage produced by detonations in chemical plant

Most of the data resulting from explosions in plant are subject to similar uncertainties in the origin of the detonation, its uniformity of propagation, the possible presence of unexpected constrictions and the response of the containment [352, 353]. Much of the experimental work on freely-expanding detonations is classified and therefore an exhaustive list of examples of damage thought to be caused by detonations is of limited value. The reader is referred to reviews quoting typical examples of recent investigations of the effects of detonations in a wide range of industrial plant, on vehicles and on buildings (see for example [354]).

In contrast, a particularly well-documented example is the destruction of a large hydroformer at Whiting, Indiana, USA, in August 1955. Reports on the investigation of the causes and effects of the explosion contain some useful advice on the use of metallurgical evidence in plotting the course of a detonation [355, 356]. Lüders lines, produced in steel stressed beyond its elastic limit, were used to trace the trajectory of the front. The advantages of external pointers to the trajectory are obvious when difficulties associated with dismantling the remains of the plant are considered. However, in this instance the plant was dismantled and the evidence from damage to internal structures confirmed the trajectory indicated by the Lüders lines. Further evidence for the position at which the detonation originated was obtained from the direction of the herring-bone patterns, associated with regions in which the structure failed in a brittle fashion. There is additional advice on the calculation of the probable velocities of fragments of plant containing burnt mixture at various temperatures and pressures, although the assumptions involved in these (such as the nature of the crack propagation and on the neglect of the expansion waves produced as the fragments accelerate) are questionable.

7.4 Experimental studies of failure resulting from detonations

There have been a number of additional studies of the effects of the normal reflection of a detonation wave from thin metallic diaphragms. Amongst these are the use of measurements of the deformation of hydraulically calibrated steel plates to estimate pressures generated by the reflection of detonation waves in mixtures of ammonia and nitrous oxide [161]. Interestingly, close agreement was claimed between the pressures measured in this way and those calculated for the reflection of a steady C–J wave in the mixture. However, there must be some reservations on the use of a suspect relationship for the pressure across the reflected wave [357]. A study of the effect of detonation waves in stoichiometric mixtures of natural gas and air reflecting from aluminium discs, showed that the discs failed dynamically at somewhat lower pressures than their static rating [358]. It was postulated that this might have been a result of vibrational fatigue. However, it seems more probable that failure to take into account the enhancement in pressure, following reflection of the front, explained the effect.

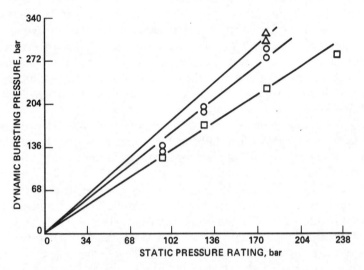

Figure 7.3 Effect of work-hardening in increasing the dynamic failure pressure of stainless steel discs. □, as received, ○ pre-pressurized by reflection of one detonation and ▽ by two detonations [359].

Luker and Leibson [359] carried out a systematic study of the failure of stainless steel, nickel, phosphor bronze and cold-rolled steel diaphragms and examined the effect of work hardening at high rates of straining. This was done by repeatedly reflecting detonations from the disc, producing pressures just below the failure level. Generally, failure occurred by shearing around the periphery of the disc. The dynamic bursting pressure (P_d) of discs of the various metals was found to be equal to or higher than the static rating of the disc (P_s), lying in the range $1.39 > P_d/P_s > 1$. Luker and Leibson's results for the work-hardening of stainless steel diaphragms in increasing the dynamic bursting pressure are illustrated in Fig. 7.3. It is in the interests of safety for pressure relief to occur at or below the expected bursting pressure of a venting diaphragm and in view of the differences between the various investigations, it is advisable dynamically to test discs which are intended for the relief of shock pressures. Again, it is important to bear in mind the consequences of possible work-hardening effects: for instance, it is advisable to replace an apparently sound bursting diaphragm, following an explosion in a plant. Further, in assessing damage from the deformation or rupture of a plate from which a detonation or shock-wave has reflected, the possibility of its having suffered work-hardening as a result of previous contained explosions should be considered.

Undoubtedly the most comprehensive study of the damaging effects of a detonation wave is that by Randall and Ginsburg [360] who examined the pressures, produced by incident fronts in $CH_4 + 2.7O_2$ mixtures, required to burst tubes of various materials. They covered the range of materials shown in Table 7.2 and examined the effect of ductility by cooling specimens to below their transition temperature for the change from ductile to brittle behaviour. A brief explanation of the arguments from which they derive bursting pressures and stresses from the ultimate tensile strengths of the materials, again shown in Table 7.2, may be helpful. By assuming that the C–J velocity of the front in the near-stoichiometric mixture is sufficiently high and the pressure profile is such that it may be treated as a suddenly applied load of

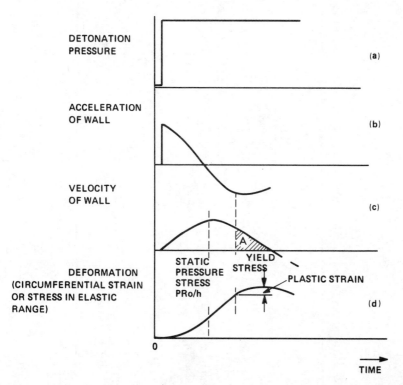

Figure 7.4 Simple model for the plastic deformation of a wall subjected to the pressure history shown in (a), area A plastically deformed [360]. For further details see text.

Table 7.2 Performance of walls of different metals subjected to an incident detonation wave [360].

Specimen	Specimen temperature (°C)	Bursting pressures (bar)		Bursting stress (bar)		% Deformation	
		Measured from detonation velocity	Estimated from tensile strength	Computed from measurements	Ultimate tensile strength	Circumferential strain in tubes	Elongation in tensile test
Machined from hot-rolled carbon–steel pipe	24	171	109	6 800	4 400	10–20	30
	–90	160–241	150	9 200	5 800	20	28
	–146	164–259	190	12 250	7 300	1	10
Cut from cold-drawn carbon–steel tubing	24	>245	230	>8 800	5 700	8	12
	–90	293	260	10 200	6 500	1–2	16
	–146	238–313	340	10 900	8 000	0.5	15
Machined from stainless steel pipe	–146	>314	306	–	12 000	28	38

uniform intensity along the length of the specimen (Fig. 7.4(a)), the radial velocity and acceleration of an element of the wall is that shown in Fig. 7.4(c) and (b). The wall stress increases sinusoidally (Fig. 7.4(d)) as the wall expands, until it balances the detonation pressure. At this position the stress is the static pressure stress and it is the position at which the pipe should eventually come to rest. However, at the static pressure stress the wall possesses its maximum radial velocity, momentarily doubling the stress, unless static pressure stresses and yield stresses coincide. By increasing the test pressures in successive experiments, Randall and Ginsburgh argue that yielding will first occur in this period of overshoot. The plateau in the history

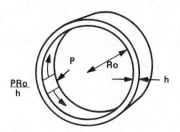

Figure 7.5 Acceleration of an element of pipe wall subjected to a constant internal pressure *P*.

of acceleration is the result of the stress in pipe wall becoming constant. The velocity of the wall consequently decreases linearly with time to zero, at which time the extension of the wall is the plastic deformation observed in the particular experiment.

A simplified analysis, analogous to that given in Equations 7.1–7.5, can be based on an element of pipe wall shown in Fig. 7.5. With the density of the wall ρ, thickness h, natural period T, Young's modulus of elasticity E, mass per unit area m, radius R_o subjected to a static pressure P, the radial motion of the wall r follows from

$$r = \frac{PR_o^2}{Eh} \qquad (7.7)$$

and the time constant of the wall is given by

$$T = 2\pi \sqrt{\left(\frac{m}{k}\right)} = 2\pi R_o \sqrt{\left(\frac{\rho}{gE}\right)} \qquad (7.8)$$

where k is the spring force and g acceleration due to gravity. In the elastic region, the radial velocity of the wall v is governed by an equation of the form

$$\frac{dv}{dt} = \frac{1}{m}(P - kr) \qquad (7.9)$$

The solution to Equation 7.9 in terms of the time elapsed from the application of the pulse t is of the form

$$r = \frac{PR_o^2}{Eh}\left[1 - \cos\frac{t}{R_o}\sqrt{\left(\frac{gE}{\rho}\right)}\right] \qquad (7.10)$$

and the circumferential stress, σ, is given by

$$\sigma = \frac{PR_o}{h}\left[1 - \cos\frac{t}{R_o}\sqrt{\left(\frac{gE}{\rho}\right)}\right] \qquad (7.11)$$

so that the time to plastic yield t_y is given in terms of the yield stress σ_y as

$$\cos\frac{t_y}{R_o}\sqrt{\left(\frac{gE}{\rho}\right)} = 1 - \frac{\sigma_y h}{PR_o} = B \qquad (7.12)$$

Hence, the velocity and acceleration at the instant of yield are

$$\left(\frac{dr}{dt}\right)_y = \frac{PR_o}{Eh}\sqrt{\left[\frac{gE}{\rho}(1 - B^2)\right]} \qquad (7.13)$$

and

$$\left(\frac{dv}{dt}\right)_y = \frac{PgB}{\rho h} \qquad (7.14)$$

so that the equation of motion changes from a sinusoidal to a linear function of time. With the assumption that yield begins in the elastic overshoot, the plastic deformation area A in Fig. 7.4(c) is obtained from the time elapsed from yield until the wall becomes stationary as the ratio of radial velocity to acceleration, so that

$$A = \frac{PR_o^2(B^2 - 1)}{2EhB} \qquad (7.15)$$

Obviously a number of the assumptions on which the analysis is based are open to criticism. Notable amongst these is the idealized pressure profile assumed to occur behind an incident detonation, the assumption that yield starts in the period of elastic overshoot, and the neglect of the effects of work-hardening in increasing strengths and of possible strain relaxation in the plastic regime. The use of more realistic pressure profiles is discussed in following sections. Again, it would be inadvisable to extrapolate from Randall and Ginsburgh's results [360] to tubes or vessels of larger diameter and consequently of longer response times and to materials in which the velocity of the stress wave is close to the C–J velocity in the gaseous mixture. An explanation of the second provision is given in later sections. Bearing in mind these uncertainties, there are a number of interesting conclusions which may be of general relevance. As Table 7.2 shows, the detonation pressure derived from the initial pressure of the mixture and the measured velocity of the front, was generally higher than the static bursting pressure which was calculated using the ultimate tensile strength of the material at the appropriate temperature in the standard expression for a thin-walled cylinder ($P_b = \sigma h / R_o$). Furthermore, the degree of plastic deformation prior to rupture apparently had no significant influence on the measured bursting pressures, with brittle failure being associated with some of the highest pressures measured. The stresses required to produce yield of the specimen were significantly higher than the static yield stress. As intuition might suggest, the number of fragments produced by failure of the tube increased as the temperature of the wall was progressively lowered below the transition value. Interestingly, a calculation of the strain rate produced by a Charpy impact test on a notched specimen showed it to be comparable with the highest values derived from measurements in their experimental set-up. Thus, a Charpy test may well produce valuable guidance on the performance of walls of different materials.

It is possible to solve the equations for the radial motion of the wall of a cylinder for a pressure pulse which more closely resembles that of a detonation. De Malherbe *et al.* [361] specified a pulse of

$$P(t) = P_i(1 - t/t_i) \text{ for } 0 < t < t_i$$

and   (7.16)

$$P(t) = 0 \qquad\qquad \text{for } t = t_i$$

where P_i is the peak pressure and t_i the duration of the pulse. Combining these with the equations of motion and retaining the previous notation leads to

$$r = \left(\frac{P_i}{T \rho h} \right) \phi \tag{7.17}$$

giving the hoop stress σ_h as

$$\sigma_h = \frac{P_i r}{h} \phi \tag{7.18}$$

where

$$\phi = 1 - t/t_i - \cos Tt + \frac{\sin Tt}{Tt_i} \qquad \text{for } 0 \leqslant t \leqslant t_i$$

and

$$\left.\phi = \left(\frac{1 - \cos Tt_i}{Tt_i}\right) \sin Tt - \left(1 - \frac{\sin Tt}{Tt_i}\right) \cos Tt \right\} \qquad (7.19)$$

$$\text{for } t > t_i$$

In analogous fashion, the axial stress σ_z on an end wall subjected to the normal reflection of a detonation can be defined as

$$\sigma_z = \left(\frac{P_r r}{2h}\right)^\phi \qquad (7.20)$$

where P_r is the peak pressure behind the reflected wave.

In a series of experiments with detonations in a 610 mm diameter stainless steel shock tube filled with stoichiometric mixtures of hydrogen and oxygen at subatmospheric pressure, hoop and axial strains were recorded by semiconductor strain gauges and pressure profiles obtained using piezoelectric pressure transducers [361]. The latter were used to deduce t_i, t_r, P_i and P_r. However, it is not clear whether the measurements of P_i and P_r subsequently used in calculating σ_h and σ_z correspond with von Neumann spike or C–J levels, although the latter seems more probable. Figure 7.6 shows a comparison of how calculated (solid line) and measured (circles and squares) values of hoop stress vary with the initial pressure of the gaseous mixture and consequently P_i. The experimental results are for two different measuring stations. Since those nearest the igniter station are somewhat lower, there must be a suggestion that a fully-developed C–J wave only occurs at distances of >4 m from the igniter. In general, the theory appears to result in tolerable predictions of the intensity of hoop and axial stresses and also an excellent description of the early stages of growth in hoop stress. However, the authors were unable to combine hoop and axial stresses, in order to define the maximum stress. Under their particular experimental conditions the hoop stresses had fallen to about 50% of their maximum amplitude before the development of axial stresses, following the reflection of the front.

Recent further extensions to the theory of response of a shell structure involving changes in the ratio of speed of waves in the gas to that in the walls are due to Brossard *et al.* [362, 363]. They examined detonations in stoichiometric mixtures of propane and oxygen (diluted with various amounts of nitrogen, $C_3H_8 + 5O_2 + ZN_2$), and their effects on tube walls of stainless steel

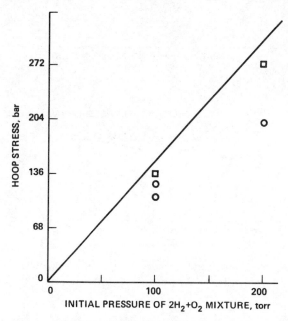

Figure 7.6   Comparison of calculated hoop stresses for a pressure history $P(t) = p_i(1 - t/t_i), 0 < t < t_i$ and $P(t) = 0, t > t_i$ with experimental measurements $\square$ 5.18 m and $\bigcirc$ 3.96 m from initiation. (After de Malherbe *et al.* [361].)

and PVC of diameters $16 \text{ mm} < d < 33 \text{ mm}$. The C–J velocity in the most heavily-diluted mixtures, 1.95 km s^{-1}, is higher than that of the stress wave in PVC, 1.75 km s^{-1}, whereas the velocity of the stress wave in stainless steel (5.3 km s^{-1}) greatly exceeds that of the C–J velocity in $C_3H_8 + 5O_2$ mixtures. Thus in PVC tubes the first event experienced at any station is the arrival of the gaseous detonation wave. Difficulties in defining a suitable law of viscoelastic behaviour precludes the development of a complete theoretical analysis for PVC. However, a number of significant experimental findings arose. In heavily-diluted mixtures of propane and oxygen PVC failed in a brittle fashion. In such cases the apparently anomalous phenomenon of more extensive damage resulting from low detonation velocities can be observed.

Figure 7.7 shows a comparison of the pressures measured at the walls of PVC tube (full line) with those calculated from deformations measured by strain gauges (points) which appear to be in reasonable agreement some $60 \,\mu s$ after the passage of the front in a tube of 17.4 mm diameter with a wall thickness of 1.25 mm. At this stage these pressures have fallen to approximately half the theoretical C–J value of 34 bar, indicated by the dashed line. Table 7.3 shows how the ratio of the pressure deduced from deformation to the C–J pressure, actually equivalent to the ratio of measured to C–J pressure, varies with the degree of dilution of the mixture and the diameter

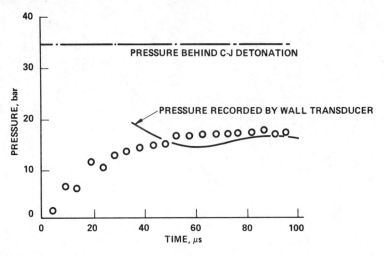

Figure 7.7 Pressures deduced from the deformation of a PVC tube subjected to a detonation in $C_3H_8 + 5O_2$, $D_{CJ} = 2.38$ km s^{-1}, after Brossard and Renard [363].

of the tube. The authors do not discuss how the effects of possible contributions to the reduction in pressure from growth of boundary layers and oxidation of the wall in the still-oxidizing products of detonation combine with those of the Taylor expansion fan. The performance of the pressure gauge itself on which the comparison is based may have some effect. The overall reduction in pressure does, however, appear to lie within the limits likely to result from a combination of these features.

The response of thin beams, flat plates and cylinders of aluminium and mild steel subjected to the normal reflection of a detonation in a mixture of methyl acetylene and propadiene has recently been examined [364]. The results are particularly noteworthy in terms of the derivation of loads from measurements of the final deformation of the structure e.g. the experiments of Randall and Ginsburgh [360] and investigations of damage produced by

Table 7.3   Effect of tube diameter and dilution of $C_3H_8 + 5O_2 + ZN_2$ mixture on the ratio of pressure calculated from deformation to C–J pressure [363].

Tube diameter (mm)	$Z = 0$	$Z = 3$	$Z = 6$	$Z = 9$
16	0.50	0.48	0.46	0.43
20	0.61	0.59	0.56	0.52
25	0.60	0.55	0.59	–
33	0.71	0.55	0.66	0.80

explosions. Thin beams securely supported at each end were observed to exhibit a series of complex shapes, as a result of the reflection of the hingeing action waves from each other and from the supports. Figure 7.8 illustrates the phenomenon with the hingeing wave moving inwards in Fig. 7.8(a) and (b) to meet in the centre in (c). If failure does not occur at this stage the reflected waves travel back towards the supports, as shown in (d) and (e). Since the deformation leaves the beam too long to pass through its original position, buckling occurs (as in (f) and (g)) and the beam eventually comes to rest, as illustrated in (h), where the buckled deformation is well below its maximum

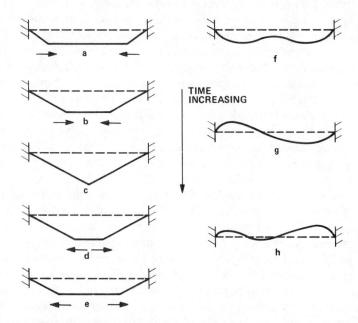

Figure 7.8   Typical response of a thin beam supported at each end to the reflection of a detonation wave [364].

value in (c). Evidently, considerable care is needed in the choice of a deformed specimen, in order to obtain reliable estimates of the peak pressure from a simple measurement of the maximum extension. In this context the damage produced in cylindrical shells by the reflection of an external detonation front is too difficult to interpret as it tends to be concentrated over approximately one quarter of the circumference. Flat square plates firmly clamped along their edges tend to behave in a more ideal fashion. In the early stages the hingeing wave moving inwards leaves the unaffected portion of the plate relatively flat. About halfway through the deflection, the central portion of the plate starts to bulge, tending towards a spherical shape. As the centre continues to distend, failure tends to occur with cracks growing along the edges of the plate close to the clamps, except at the corners where the crack moves diagonally across.

7.5 Concluding remarks

While a full understanding of the mechanisms of failure and of the type of damage associated with the loads imposed by a detonation is obviously of high importance to the safe design of equipment containing flammable mixtures, the foregoing makes it clear that they are objectives unlikely to be attained in the near future. In particular, in investigations of incidents, it is not surprising that estimates of the effective pressures, made from measurements of deformation at which similar pressures might be supposed to exist, vary over a wide range. In the author's experience factors of up to ten are not uncommon. It is difficult to give cogent but generally-applicable advice, either to the investigator of damage caused by an explosion or to a designer attempting to ensure the effects of a detonation are contained. It is worth emphasizing that nearly all available information has been obtained with mixtures of fuel and oxidant of close to stoichiometric composition. Thus, the effects of wide variations in local pressures due to the non-planarity of fronts in marginally-detonable mixtures have been minimized. Furthermore, little consideration has been paid to the effects of internal structures in these laboratory experiments. The enhancement in local peak pressures produced by Mach and regular reflection at such obstructions or in bends and junctions, can play a dominant role in determining damage to plant. This effect can be reinforced by partial quenching, followed by explosive re-establishment of the incident front.

Bearing in mind these provisions, available experimental evidence does not indicate greater degrees of damage to plant from the dynamic loads imposed by detonations than would be predicted from its static rating. It is possible to account for this apparent anomaly, for instance in terms of enhanced work-hardening of metals in high rates of strain. However, the bases of such explanations are sufficiently tenuous to suggest caution in the general application of the equivalence of the effects of static with detonation type loads to the complex geometries occurring in plant.

It has often been suggested that some improvement on the performance of plant subjected to internal explosions can be expected when ductile materials of construction are used. However, it should be noted that the only available experimental information on the relative performance of ductile and brittle materials indicates that ductility has little effect on the dynamic bursting pressure. It may be dangerous to attempt a sweeping generalization from the limited data. The prevention or significant reduction in fragmentation with more ductile materials does result in a significant reduction in the hazards of injury to personnel. As a palliative measure, it is evidently necessary to attempt to restrain or capture potential fragments.

8

Prevention and mitigation of detonations

8.1 Introductory remarks

A number of factors mitigate against the production of a well-balanced account of the procedures available for the control of detonations. The minimal conditions required for a detonation wave are the simultaneous occurrence of a flammable mixture and an ignition source for mixtures of fuel and oxidant, or an excursion in the working pressure into the critical regime plus ignition source for an exothermically self-decomposing fuel. However, a detailed and general discussion of the avoidance of such conditions in plant is evidently outside the scope of the present text. Notwithstanding this, it is useful to draw attention to the additional potential source of ignition in two-phase systems which involves the possibility of the particles or droplets becoming charged during some stage in their processing, for example during size-reduction, with a resultant local and intense electrical discharge to an earthed portion of the plant.

The inhibition and quenching of flames of normal burning velocity has been intensively studied and the mechanisms governing the action of certain classes of inhibitors identified. Thus halogen-containing compounds, products of their pyrolysis, sulphur dioxide, etc. act by catalysing the recombination or destruction of atomic species such as hydrogen or oxygen atoms and hydroxyl radicals which are responsible for the chain-branching reaction steps essential for the flame. For instance, reaction steps such as

$$H^{\bullet} + Cl^{\bullet} + M \rightarrow HCl + M \qquad (8.1)$$

compete with chain-branching reactions of the type

$$H^{\bullet} + O_2 \rightarrow HO^{\bullet} + O^{\bullet} \qquad (8.2)$$

to reduce the above equilibrium concentrations of atomic species and radicals characteristic of a normal flame. The mechanisms involved in inhibition by particles of sodium and potassium salts of organic acids are less clear-cut, making it difficult to predict the relative efficiency of such inhibitors. It may well be that their action involves a combination of energy removal during their heating and endothermic decomposition with chemical inhibition associated with the decomposition products of carbon dioxide and the atoms of alkali metals. Inevitably, the resultant literature is too wide-ranging to attempt more than a summary here. Full details are contained in standard texts on combustion [8, 365]. There is some useful information on halogen-containing additives [366] and a helpful comparison of the relative effectiveness of a variety of metals derived from the pyrolysis of their salts with organic acids [367]. It is also possible readily to quench flames of low velocities by conventional forms of flame trap. These are described in Section 8.2.

A logical approach to the control of detonations starts with a description of methods of quenching the initial flame, followed by a section on methods of preventing the early stages of its acceleration by pressure-relieving devices. This is an area which has been intensively studied so that there is an extensive literature covering work on the venting of flames in clouds of dust and on the venting of gaseous explosions [368–370]. In the interests of brevity we have attempted no more than a short survey of the main features of practical interest and a brief reference to features which are not normally considered. Following sections deal with the suppression of a flame–shock complex, produced by an accelerating flame, and the quenching of detonations travelling at uniform C–J velocities. Frequently similar quenching agents are effective throughout all stages of the initiation of a detonation. However, the decreasing times available for suppression as the flame accelerates towards C–J velocities result in more stringent requirements of the preventative measures. Finally, one technique suitable for the mitigation of an explosion of an unconfined vapour cloud is discussed.

This choice of presentation does not anticipate a series of devices on the plant to deal with each stage in the development of a detonation; rather that every reasonable precaution be taken to avoid the simultaneous occurrence of a flammable mixture and a source of ignition. Some form of risk analysis should be applied to the specific plant, in order to determine the most appropriate second line of defence. For example, the malfunction of equipment designed to gasify coal dust in oxygen may result in the unavoidable occurrence of a detonable suspension and an ignition source in high-velocity flows through pipelines. In such an instance, it may be necessary to ensure that the preventative measures are capable of quenching a C–J detonation.

At first sight it would appear that the suppression of a steady C–J detonation in stoichiometric mixtures of fuel and oxidant is the most severe test of a quenching procedure. Certainly, most suppression systems have been tested using such mixtures. However, some notes of caution are appropriate. The high velocity of sound in hydrogen means that C–J velocities steadily increase as a mixture of hydrogen with oxidant becomes progressively more fuel-rich, so that times available for suppression progressively decrease with increasing fuel content in the mixture. Again in practice, the mixture most likely to be produced in the event of a failure is one close to the lower limit of detonability. The effects of the distribution of the localized areas of high pressure and high rates of energy release associated with near-limit mixtures must be carefully assessed. For instance, the length of a detonation arrester must be many times that of the characteristic length of the transverse structure of the wave, say ≥ 100 times the spacing of the transverse fronts for a mixture of the given composition, pressure and temperature.

Although not all the features of the interactions of detonation waves in fuel-lean mixtures are understood, it is worth emphasizing that, in general, accidents leading to formation of a fuel-lean rather than fuel-rich mixture are likely to have less dire consequences. With a fuel-rich mixture, the danger of a detonation evidently persists throughout the period of dilution from fuel-rich to fuel lean. During this phase there is the additional danger that the detonation is formed in a close-to-stoichiometric mixture, resulting in a leading shock of persistently high strength.

8.2 Inhibition of flames of normal burning velocity

In general, the various chemical processes which the fuel eventually experiences will preclude the permanent presence of an inhibitor. Consequently, the usual practice is to trigger the injection by a signal from some form of flame-detector. With long runs of pipeline it is advisable to consider the installation of a number of detectors and possibly more than one injection station. With an array of detectors it is possible to process the signals electronically to give the direction in which the flame is travelling, and thus to trigger the appropriate injector. A typical arrangement is shown in Fig. 8.1. The optimum choice of position for the detectors requires a prediction of the most probable site of ignition. In general the direction of flame propagation will be that of the original flow, but at low rates of flow the possibility of flashback always exists.

In the early stages of the development of an explosion, the velocities of both contained and uncontained flames are quite low. Burning velocities of mixtures of fuel with air are typically ≤ 1 m s^{-1}, with hydrogen–air mixtures about an order of magnitude higher. Replacing air by oxygen results in an increase by a factor of 10. Allowing a typical expansion ratio $\epsilon \leq 10$, flame velocities likely to be encountered under plant-fault conditions are generally not much greater than 10 m s^{-1}. Thus, there is usually ample time for the processes of injection and quenching of the flame, even by relatively inefficient inhibitors, such as a curtain of water droplets. Assuming the injector and flame detector are 5 m apart, 0.5 s is available for producing a water fog before arrival of the flame. There is little difficulty in designing the injector to produce a fog of at least 5 m in length, so that ≥ 0.5 s is available for the quenching process. For faster burning mixtures such as hydrogen–air or mixtures of hydrocarbons with oxygen, it is advisable to use a more efficient inhibitor, such as a halogenated hydrocarbon.

A wide variety of materials can be used to quench flames travelling at low velocities. They range from inert powders or water droplets which act by the physical mechanism of removal of energy, to highly efficient catalysts of radical recombination reactions. They include powdered salts of organic acids, carbonates and bicarbonates which may well combine the extraction of energy from the flame with the production of carbon dioxide, a tolerably effective quenching agent. Arguably the most widely used powder inhibitor is mono-ammonium phosphate. Other additives such as CrO_2Cl_2, $Pb(C_2H_5)_4$ and $Fe(CO)_5$ are even more efficient than halogenated hydrocarbons and apparently function via the formation of the metal oxide in the flame, which

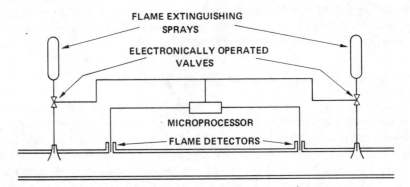

Figure 8.1 Typical arrangement for triggered suppression of a flame propagating in either direction in a pipeline.

again catalyses recombination reactions [371]. Halogenated hydrocarbons are generally used in commercially-supplied suppression equipment. As liquids they are readily introduced as high-pressure sprays. However, they suffer from the disadvantage that the products of decomposition are both toxic and corrosive. There are similar advantages and disadvantages associated with the use of the other additives listed. It may be that a final choice should be based on economic grounds, taking into consideration the costs of an accidental triggering of the injection system which may be up to £1,000 for long pipelines of large diameter and large reactor vessels. In this context single commercial injectors can deliver 1–10 kg of inhibitor, considerably in excess of the amount which, if uniformly dispersed, would be required from a consideration of flammability limits. On the grounds of cost, the use of water sprays deserves serious consideration.

Up to this stage the suppression of flames has been considered in terms of mixtures confined in pipelines. However, preventative measures can be used on cylindrical or spherical reaction vessels. The largest dimension of these will be much less than the length of a typical pipeline, so that the combined time for injection and quenching is reduced. Generally, precautions against central ignition (potentially the most dangerous situation) will be taken, so that only one detector should be required although it may be advisable to install more than a single extinguishing spray with large vessels. These should ensure a uniform distribution of the extinguishant and protect against the effects of non-symmetrically spreading flames, caused by effects such as buoyancy.

For the protection of pipelines it is possible to incorporate conventional flame arresters. These can be in the form of a number of metallic gauzes, sintered metallic discs, a honeycomb metal packing or a spirally wound composite of straight and crimped metallic strip. The appropriate choice depends on the allowable pressure drop across the arrester. Assuming equivalent efficiency per unit length of the arrester in removing energy from the flame and burnt gases, the wound crimped strip will generally result in the lowest drop in pressure. Usually a length of about a metre is sufficient and the penalty of the imposed pressure drop may well be counterbalanced by reduced requirements for maintenance compared with triggered extinguishing systems. It is worth noting that the siting of arresters can be crucial, as in the later stages of an explosion they may act as generators of turbulence and consequently enhance the acceleration of the flame. Finally, on account of potential blockage, their use is generally precluded for two-phase mixtures.

8.3 Venting in the early stages of an explosion

An alternative approach to suppressing the initial flame is to prevent its acceleration and the generation of an explosion by some form of pressure relief. This is generally a less expensive solution than flame suppression. Consequently, extensive efforts have gone into studies of various devices for the relief of pressure and their optimum siting for mixtures with a wide range of laminar burning velocities. There is an extensive literature on the subject, covering the use of bursting diaphragms and hinged and spring-loaded explosion doors. The practical aspects of venting of both gaseous and dust explosions have been extensively studied and there is a range of excellent reviews [372, 373]. A recent publication gives detailed recommendations for the venting of explosions of dust clouds [370]. However, much of the information on which these are based comes from experimental and theoretical work on the relief of pressure in compact vessels (length/diameter $\gg 3$) in which symmetry of flow exists throughout the process [374]. In general a single vent is fitted to the vessel to be protected, so that flows become unsymmetrical as soon as it opens. One consequence is that the outflow from largish vessels can result in the production of turbulence, localized acceleration of the flame and the generation of a second peak in pressure. Figure 8.2 shows a typical pressure history from a vented explosion in a large vessel, with turbulent flow through a single vent [375]. The second peak is some four times the initial vented peak, occurring just after opening of the vent, and points to the dangers in basing a design on the opening pressure of the vent. The subsequent oscillations in pressure can be accounted for by the reflection of expansion and pressure waves within the vessel leading to the production of steep pressure gradients [376]. There is some guidance available on the features influencing venting under such circumstances, and this draws attention to the potential dangers of the abrupt reversals in pressure gradients coupling with the natural frequency of the vessel [377].

A useful summary of venting precautions required of a lengthy pipeline in which bends, junctions and changes in cross-section are likely to feature, has been published [378]. Among its important recommendations is a requirement for measures of pressure relief both before and after every change in

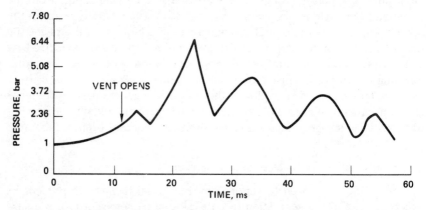

Figure 8.2 Growth in explosive pressure brought about by turbulent outflow from a vent (after Harris and Briscoe [375]).

shape or direction of the pipe. For mixtures with laminar burning velocities ≤ 3 m s^{-1} in straight pipelines of ratio of length to diameter $(L/d) > 30$, pressure relief at intervals which depend on the ratio of the area of the vent to that of the cross-section of the pipe (K) is recommended. Table 8.1 shows the relationship between K, the recommended spacing of vents and the maximum pressure. It is important to consider how the hot gases from vents may be discharged without causing potential hazard to personnel and without imposing severe penalties in the efficiency of pressure relief. The safe siting of the large number of vents for a long pipeline of small diameter may well pose a severe problem. In this context, it should be noted that additional ductwork intended to channel the burnt gases to safety can impair venting. A doubling in the maximum pressure developed in a vented explosion for every five diameters of duct attached to the relief device has been suggested [379].

The original procedures recommended for pressure relief in the early stages of an explosion were based on experiments with gaseous mixtures [380].

Table 8.1 Recommended spacing of pressure relief for pipelines $L/d > 30$ containing mixtures $S_u \leq 3$ m s^{-1} [378].

K	Recommended spacing	P_{max} $(kN\,m^{-2})$
1	60 d	16.54
2	30 d	13.09
4	20 d	11.03
8	15 d	10.34

However, it has been suggested that they are also applicable to dust clouds, providing they are based on the equivalence of burning velocities [381]. Further valuable sources of reference of venting of explosions of clouds of dust are given in various books [368–370] and in texts on the venting of gaseous explosions [382].

In general, vents of the type described are only likely to be favoured in systems with low working pressures, say a maximum of a few bar. Higher working pressures impose severe problems on the design of efficient arrangements for pressure relief. For instance, there are those associated with coping with normal excursions in the working pressure. The increasing thickness of the walls of vessels makes it difficult to design vents of sufficiently short opening times. Thus, other precautions must be considered.

8.4 Quenching of flame–shock complexes

Most of the preventative measures appropriate to flames of low velocity can be modified to remain effective at the stage at which the flame has accelerated to close-to-sonic velocity, when first a shock is formed. However, a ratio of sonic velocity to that of the flame in the initial stages of the development ≤ 30 means that the times to effect measures of control and subsequently to suppress the deflagration are drastically reduced. A notable example is the German chemical industry's use of various ceramic packings in pipelines carrying pure acetylene at high pressures during the early 1940s. The pipelines were designed to contain the highest pressure that could be generated by a deflagration in acetylene (about 10 bar), and the packings proved extremely effective in preventing a transition to detonation.

In one instance, advantage has been taken of the properties of the leading shock to initiate suppression of the following flame front. In mine galleries, trays containing limestone dust or water supported on readily dislodged shelves, spaced along the length of the gallery roof can be toppled by the shocked flow, dispersing the inerting material in the unburnt mixture ahead of the flame [383]. However, although such devices are highly successful in quenching the flame, they do not alleviate the pressures behind the leading shock. The subsequent attenuation of the leading front can only occur through the very slow processes associated with viscous drag at the walls. This technique does not appear to have found any application to pipelines at risk from a potentially flammable gaseous mixture. This is probably connected with difficulties in inspecting the state of such devices in a conventional pipeline. Again, there is the possibility that badly sited barriers create additional turbulence, leading to further acceleration of the flame. The latter feature should discourage the application of conventional flame arresters to the later stages of a pipeline in which it is possible for a detonation to form.

Special precautions are required to attenuate the pressures behind the leading shock. The most effective method of doing so is the introduction of a large and abrupt expansion in cross-section. However, it will be recalled that the interaction of the shock and the expansion waves created around the rim of the area change is a relatively slow process, and some five to ten diameters of the inlet are required before the shock at the axis of symmetry decays to a sound wave [294, 295]. A possible solution is a series of transverse slits along the length of pipeline potentially subject to a detonation. Since attenuation of the detonation front is a relatively slow process, it is difficult to specify the optimum spacing and width of slits [384].

Flames associated with a leading shock in gaseous mixtures, clouds of dusts and aerosols can be quenched by a wide variety of additives. In particular there have been extensive studies of flame-quenching in both vessels and pipelines, the length and diameter of which approach the maximum values likely to be encountered in plant [370]. The reference contains a wealth of detail on the design and performance of commercially available flame-suppressant systems. Somewhat surprisingly it gives little consideration to the subsequent interactions of the leading shock; thus it is appropriate here only to draw attention to such neglected features.

There is evidence that larger quantities of suppressants are required in the later stages of an explosion. Table 8.2 shows a comparison of the amounts of bromochlorodifluoromethane (BCF) required to suppress the later stages of a coal dust–air explosion in a 1.2 m diameter, 68 m long explosion gallery [181] with those required for the earlier stages of a similar explosion in a 0.15 m diameter, 3.6 m long tube [385]. In addition to the order of magnitude increase in the dimensions of the explosion gallery, a captive rocket was used as the source of ignition, resulting in pronounced acceleration of the flame and consequent growth in pressure, shown by the pressure recording in the absence of BCF in Fig. 8.3. Following the injection of BCF the growth of explosive pressures is effectively quenched in about 0.2 s. Table 8.2 also indicates that carbon tetrachloride and BCF are equally effective in quenching the growth in pressure but that up to four times the amount of inhibitor is required in the later stages of the explosion. It is difficult to find such a clear-cut example in gaseous explosions. However, the nominal concentrations delivered by commercial extinguishing systems for gaseous systems indicate that they behave in a similar fashion.

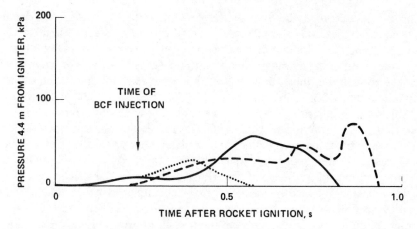

Figure 8.3 Inhibition of a developed coal-dust–air explosion by addition of BCF. —— coal-dust at closed end only, BCF absent; – – – coal-dust at closed end and 16.8 m, BCF absent; ··· coal dust at closed end and 16.8 m, BCF injection at 8.5 m. (After Rae and Thompson [181].)

Table 8.2 Comparison of quantities of suppressants required to quench the early stages [385] and the later stages [181] of a coal dust–air explosion.

	Coal concentration as a function of a stoichiometric mixture of coal dust with air	*% (mass) BCF*	*% (mass) CCl_4*
Early stage of	0.75	21	
explosion [385]	1.00	18	
	1.25	14	
Later stage of	1.30	59	57
explosion [181]	3.20	15	17–23

Apart from the special case of air–coal-dust explosions in mine galleries, it is unusual to design control measures specifically for the flame–shock stage of the explosion. Normally, designs for the injection of flame inhibitors are based on quenching the early stages of the flame. Thus, it is important to be aware of measures which can be taken to control detonation waves.

8.5 Suppression of detonations

The presence of the sonic C–J plane at some ill-defined distance behind the leading shock restricts measures to control detonations travelling at uniform C–J velocities to ones directly influencing the leading front. This is because the effects of an expansion fan generated behind the sonic plane cannot influence the leading front. Thus, preventative measures must be based on an abrupt expansion in the area of the containment. Although it has been suggested that a series of transverse slits might prove satisfactory in the early stages of the development of a detonation [384], their width, dictated by a consideration of the meeting of the expansion waves at the axis of symmetry, would be such that they can be regarded as abrupt expansions. Our growing understanding of the nature of the critical diameter for an abrupt expansion [118] and its relationship with the spacing of transverse waves on the leading shock has been described in Chapter 6. This can readily be used as a basis for quenching, by designing pipelines to be of a diameter below the critical value and incorporating an abrupt expansion at an appropriate site. However, it requires either a knowledge of the critical diameter or the spacing of transverse waves for the mixture most likely to be encountered in the containment. It may be difficult to predict the optimum position of the expansion. Further practical difficulties may arise from the pressure drops and non-steady flow conditions existing in such an arrester during normal operation of the plant [386].

Table 8.3 Experimental values for area increase, length of flame arrester and position for quenching detonations in stoichiometric mixtures of town gas with air [47].

Inlet diameter	Measured detonation velocity	Diameter of expanded pipe	Length of flame arrester	Distance between area change and arrester
(cm)	(km s^{-1})	(cm)	(cm)	(cm)
2.5	1.65	8.9	3.2	2.5–7.0
3.8	–	17.8	3.8	5.1–20.3
5.1	1.89	17.8	3.8	7.6–22.9
7.6	–	35.6	4.4	15.2–38.1
10.2	1.98	35.6	4.4	22.9–61.0

Notwithstanding these difficulties, abrupt expansions in area combined with conventional flame arresters have been used to check detonations. In general, an arbitrary choice of the ratio of outlet to inlet areas appears to have been made. A series of experiments showed that detonations in a stoichiometric mixture of town gas with air could be successfully suppressed by the combination of an expansion and flame trap constructed of a spirally-wound, crimped metal, sited on the expanded tube [47]. The results, given in Table 8.3, show that the detonation is arrested when the ratio of the diameter of the expanded pipe to the inlet pipe is about four, for pipeline diameters up to 10 cm. Table 8.3 includes experimental measurements for the required length of the flame arrester, its optimum position to prevent re-establishment and the variation in detonation velocity with the diameter of the tube. It is unfortunate that there is no information about the spacing of transverse waves on a detonation in a stoichiometric mixture of town gas with air at atmospheric pressure, so its relationship with the range of diameter of pipes tested remains unclear. What is apparent however, is the increase in severity of the duties of the flame arrester, marked by the increase in length, required to deal with the higher detonation velocities in the pipes of larger diameter.

A variety of flame arresters have been combined successfully with an expansion in area. For instance, discs made from a foamed nickel-chromium alloy and aluminium ballast rings have been shown to quench detonations propagating at velocities of about 1.8 km s^{-1} in mixtures of petroleum vapour

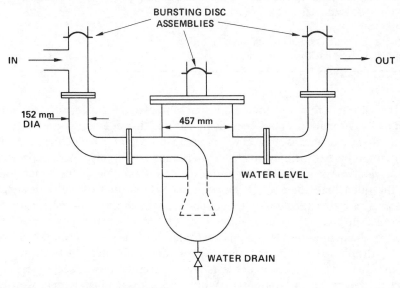

Figure 8.4   Water trap arrester [48].

with air in a 15.3 cm diameter stainless steel tube [48]. The arresters were used in conjunction with an area expansion ratio of four. The study also demonstrated that a conventional water-trap type arrester, shown schematically in Fig. 8.4, was effective. The ratio of diameters of outlet to inlet for this is about three. Table 8.4 gives a brief description of the number of experiments in which the arresters performed satisfactorily, which lends some confidence to their effectiveness. The final column gives the pressure drop associated with the combined arrester and area increase under steady-state conditions. Further experiments with detonations in mixtures of butane with air in a 7.6 cm diameter tube confirm the effectiveness in quenching of a doubling in diameter of the pipe combined with a packing of aluminium rings [387]. Unfortunately, there is no direct information on spacing of transverse fronts for either petroleum vapour–air or butane–air mixtures. From evidence from other hydrocarbons in the alkane series the spacing is likely to be at least 1 cm, so that, at least in the latter case, it is likely that the pipeline was below the critical diameter.

Table 8.4 Commercially available quenching devices used to suppress detonations in gaseous mixtures of petroleum and air [48].

Detonation arrester	Number of successful tests	Pressure drop $(kN\,m^{-2})$
Shand and Jurs spiral-wound crimped aluminium ribbon	9	0.15
Whessoe 80-grade retimet foamed metal	3	0.24
Water trap	5	1.66
Vertically-stacked bed of aluminium ballast rings	5	0.05
Linde hydraulic back-pressure valve	6	2.03

It is also possible to combine a water spray with an expansion in area to control a detonation. It has been demonstrated that detonations in mixtures of methane and air travelling at velocities up to 1.8 km s^{-1} in pipelines of 0.6 m in diameter are invariably quenched by a combination of an increase in area with water sprays [358]. However, there is no information on the dimensions of the quenching chamber. It has also been found that carefully designed systems of water injection halt a detonation without the requirement for an increase in area. Table 8.5 summarizes the amounts of water needed to control the detonation. No details are available of the size distribution of the water droplets or of the duration, distribution and extent of the sprays – evidently, further experimental tests are required to answer such questions and to determine the optimum conditions for quenching. It may well be possible to reduce the minimum requirement of water from that used in these experiments.

Table 8.5 Inhibition of gaseous detonations by water jets only [358].

Injection system	Number of successful tests	Mass of water / Mass of fuel
2 rings of jets, 0.3 m apart	4	16.7
2 rings of jets, 1.5 m apart	2	22.0
	2	7.0
	2	5.8

It is unfortunate that the one fundamental study of suppression of detonation waves in which careful attention was paid to the relationship between the dimensions of the quenching device and the spacing of transverse waves ended in a negative result [388]. Thus, it was found to be impossible to quench detonations, velocity 2.3 km s^{-1}, in stoichiometric mixtures of propane and oxygen using a honeycomb of steel blades spaced 6 mm apart (some two to three times the spacing of the transverse waves), with the arrester in a pipe of unchanged cross-section. It is possible to argue that either decreasing the spacing of the blades to approach that of the transverse fronts or incorporating an expansion in area would have resulted in successful suppression. However, the paper suggests that quenching only occurs when the velocity of the leading front is decreased sufficiently for the temperature in the flow behind it to be low enough to prevent ignition. This is probably an over-simplistic approach, in view of the complex and localized nature of the deceleration of the wave as it travels through the various sections of the honeycomb.

Table 8.6 Weight and surface area of inhibitor required to suppress an established detonation in $CH_4 + 2O_2 + N_2$ mixtures [45].

Inhibitor	Surface area per unit weight	Weight for suppression (g)	Surface area (m^2)
Silica	395	0.825	0.326
Potassium chloride	279	2.15	0.60
Potassium bicarbonate	415	0.835	0.347
Potassium oxalate	522	0.920	0.48
Potassium bitartrate	765	0.46	0.352
Sodium bitartrate	740	0.93	0.69

It will be recalled that a number of gaseous additives have been shown to reduce the detonability limits of confined stoichiometric mixtures of hydrogen and oxygen. In addition, a variety of powders have been found to quench confined detonations in $CH_4 + 2O_2 + N_2$ mixtures [45]. Table 8.6 lists the powders tested, their surface area ($10 < d < 20\ \mu$m) and the mass and derived surface area required for successful quenching. Because of the pronounced effects of the properties of the particles in governing the uniformity of dispersion of the cloud, some caution must be observed in attempting to deduce mechanisms from their relative efficiencies. The difference in effectiveness of potassium and sodium bitartrate points to some form of chemical influence. However, chemically the relative inert silica particles perform better, in marked contrast to the relative effectiveness in suppressing normal

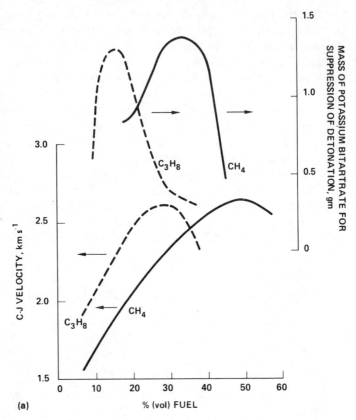

Figure 8.5 (a), (b) Suppression of confined detonations by powders (after Laffite and Bouchet [45]).

flames. It is possible to infer that the controlling parameter is the surface area of the additive. Figures 8.5(a) and (b) show the mass of potassium bitartrate required to quench detonations in mixtures with high and low C–J velocities respectively and how detonation velocities and amounts of suppressant vary with the composition of the mixture. The C–J velocity itself has surprisingly little effect on the mass of suppressants needed, but the largest quantities are required for mixtures approaching the stoichiometric composition. The actual concentrations used are high. Thus, a typical minimum concentration calculated assuming uniform distribution throughout the tube is as high as 50 kg m^{-3}.

8.6 Mitigating the effects of detonations

Frequently the walls of straight sections of pipework of small diameter are sufficiently thick to withstand the effects of a detonation without incurring

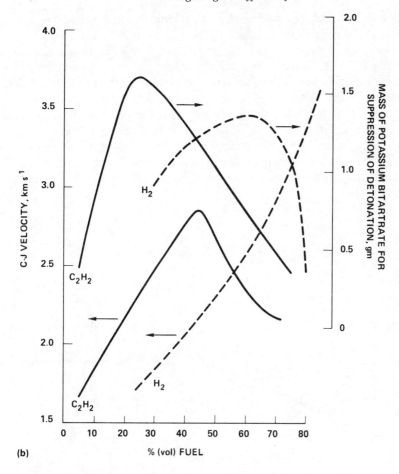

(b)

severe damage. Failure occurs in regions such as bends and junctions where still higher pressures are generated by the partial reflection of the incident wave. The end of a pipeline subjected to an internal detonation is particularly at risk, following the normal reflection over its whole surface of the incident front. The possibility of fitting either end caps which can be explosively destroyed just prior to the arrival of the incident front or triggered fast-acting valves in the end plate has been considered [370]. The system must be designed so that the flame detector responds to the explosion before its transition to a detonation, and the end vent is activated just before the fully-developed detonation arrives. Should the end vent open too early, there is a grave danger that a resultant outflow of unburnt mixture generating turbulence may create a detonation which would not otherwise be formed. There can be no hard and fast general rules for the design of the activation procedures for such a vent. This becomes clear from consideration of a pipeline in which the probability of an ignition source occurring at any position is similar along its length.

The procedures described so far generally imply alleviation measures which are applied to a detonation in some form of containment. A procedure which is appropriate to either the later stages of a deflagration in which a shock has formed or the detonation of an unconfined cloud of vapour has been suggested [49]. It is based on the experimental observation that it is possible to utilize the acoustic mismatch across an interface between gases of low and high sonic velocities to reduce significantly the strength of the wave transmitted through the medium of high sonic velocity. This leads to the possibility of triggering the formation of a helium barrier on the escape of the vapour, to

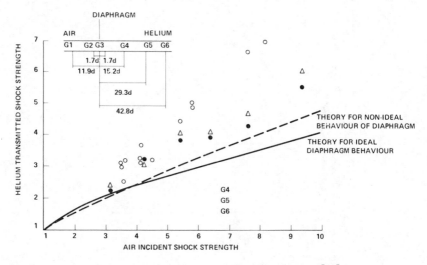

Figure 8.6   Attenuation of a shock wave at a slow–fast interface [49].

protect buildings against the effect of a detonation of the cloud. As the detonation travels into the concentration gradient of increasingly higher content of helium, the leading shock should rapidly attenuate and the following reaction zones should be quenched by the inerting effect of helium. The experiments were carried out in a channel in which helium was separated from air by a diaphragm. The incident wave in air was consequently reflected from this, so that the front transmitted into the helium was initially overdriven. Figure 8.6 shows how this overdriven wave decays as it travels through the helium, to approach the values predicted by an analysis of refraction of a shock at an acoustic interface [336]. Such an encouraging result suggests that there may be scope for other measures such as a triggered curtain of sprays, or more permanent ones such as a liquid foam or possibly a foamed plastic.

8.7 Concluding remarks

There is a wide range of measures available for the control of the various stages in the development of a detonation. Certain of these, such as triggered injection of flame inhibitors, are effective in quenching all stages, including a steady C–J detonation. However, as the duties of the quenching system become more onerous as the stage of detonation is approached, larger concentrations of inhibitor and faster acting injection systems are required. The choice and design of appropriate protective procedures depends on the type and dimensions of plant, the nature of the potentially-detonable medium and the probability of occurrence and strength of ignition sources. It is only possible here to draw attention to some general features which influence this choice.

In the absence of energetic sources of initiation detonations are more probable in pipelines than in compact reaction vessels. However, such distances allow sufficient time for effective measures of suppression. There are few, if any, examples of detonations in clouds of flammable dust in air in industrial equipment. Consequently, such plant is only built to withstand overpressures less than 1 bar, and typical grain storage and transport facilities are fitted with vents to deal with the effects of the early stages of flame propagation. In some instances it may be possible to envisage the formation of an energetic initiator, for instance a shock created by the rupture of a vessel initially at high pressures. In this case, a rapidly-triggered fast-acting quenching system is evidently necessary. Similar measures are appropriate for processes in which the oxygen content is higher than that in air. It is also worth noting that a number of different control measures may be fitted to the various components in a chemical plant. Thus vessels at the origin of the process line, e.g. size reduction equipment, may be fitted with vents. At this stage there is little danger from the direct initiation of a detonation. Pipelines transporting the products at a later stage in the process may be protected by triggered extinguishers or may be of sufficient strength to contain the effects of a detonation.

9

Concluding recommendations

9.1 Introductory remarks

Chapter 1 described in general terms some of the problems involved in the appropriate choice of design criteria for plants at potential risk from the effects of a detonation. They were shown to originate from the lack of a comprehensive theory describing the complex system of shocks and reaction zones comprising a steady detonation front. Consequently, attempts to describe changes in the structure of the front, brought about by variations in the properties of the detonable media or by the interaction of the wave with changes in its confinement, are generally interpreted in terms of inappropriate unidimensional concepts. The increasingly ready availability of powerful numerical techniques for predicting the response of complex structures to dynamic loads [43, 44], with their consequent requirements for accurate descriptions of pressure histories and their variation with properties of the medium and its confinement, emphasize the need for a consistent approach, based on the multi-dimensionality of real detonation fronts. That which has been adopted here should serve to identify with some degree of accuracy the range of local pressures generated by detonations in readily detonable media and, less precisely, those likely to exist in more marginal media. However, in their role as yardsticks for measuring the performance of multi-dimensional theories, such numerical treatments of structural response highlight the need for a better description of local temporal variations in pressure. The need for further work in this and other areas on the variation in the local properties of the front is described in fuller detail in Section 9.5.

Some caution is necessary in contemplating the development of more comprehensive theories of multi-dimensional waves: for instance it has been noted that some of the processes involved in the initiation of a detonation [207] and its interactions with changes in confinement [296] may be stochastic in nature. Consequently, although further work should result in more precise definitions of the effects of changes in the media and its confinement on the pressure histories, it is unlikely to allow a matching of a particular pressure profile with a unique location. Any resultant model is unlikely to predict a complete list of detonable media, together with the necessary experimental conditions for detonability. Although Chapter 4 contains as comprehensive as possible a list, there are almost certainly omissions of less common fuels and oxidants at initial pressures and temperatures close to ambient, and probably of a wider range of fuels and oxidants at elevated pressures and temperatures. It is therefore worth emphasizing the philosophy (outlined in Chapter 4) of ensuring that appropriate precautions are observed with any media known to react exothermically and with those where the molar ratio of products to that of reactants is much greater than unity.

The design of chemical plant, at risk from the effects of a detonation, has been assessed historically on the basis of a comparison of the pressures, predicted by unidimensional theories, with the slowly-applied pressure which the plant can safely withstand. The deficiencies implicit in this approach are readily recognizable. Thus, the pressures predicted by unidimensional theories are well below the local pressures produced by real waves. Also, when assessing potential damage, the approach neglects the probable differences between stress–strain relationships at the high rates of strain imposed by a detonation and those produced by slowly-applied loads. In the same context, it takes no account of the relationship between the shape of the applied pressure profile and the response time of the structure. Fortunately in general, the pressures given by unidimensional theories for fronts propagating in media at, or above, atmospheric pressure are too high to be accommodated in all but straight runs of open-ended and small diameter pipelines of normal wall thickness. This has led to the widespread application of solutions, based on the adoption of measures to prevent or rapidly to quench detonations. This is despite the fact that the limited number of experiments [359, 360] on the damaging effects of detonations suggest that the historical criterion is indeed a safe one. It should be recalled that these tests were performed with stoichiometric mixtures of fuel and oxidant, so that departures in pressure from those of idealized theories were minimized.

Chapter 8 covered in detail specific measures for quenching incipient and established detonations, and for the relief of damagingly high pressures. However, at this stage it is appropriate to emphasize some of the more general features, which can either be incorporated in the design of the plant or taken in operating procedures, both to reduce the risks of the formation of a detonation wave and to mitigate its effects. The most obvious of these is the need for stringent precautions against the occurrence of possible ignition sources for flames and more energetic sources which could lead to the direct initiation of detonation. The hazards associated with electrical and chemical sparks, as produced for instance by the reaction of aluminium with iron oxide, are widely recognized. Occasionally however, explosions have been attributed to the presence of much less common sources. For example, the possible presence of detonators and mining explosives have been considered in investigations of explosions in size comminution equipment. Particularly stringent precautions against the possible discharge of static electricity are necessary in the case of dust clouds and aerosols.

Further features of good design practice consist in minimizing the diameter and length of pipelines and avoiding abrupt changes in shape and cross-section, especially those which present to an incipient shock front a compressive surface. In terms of the possibility of a leak from a chemical plant or storage facility, forming an unconfined or partly-confined cloud of vapour, it is obviously desirable to minimize the inventory of fuel being processed or stored. Consequently, there is a degree of conflict between the economies of large-scale processing and the cost penalties of increased safety. However there is some scope for compromise in, for instance, the use of numbers of small storage vessels to replace a single unit with a large inventory of fuel. The former can be fitted with cut-off valves for automatic isolation in the event of a sudden drop in pressure. Similarly, compressors can be equipped with control systems resulting in their automatic shut-down in the event of sudden decompression in equipment downstream.

It is generally agreed that turbulence promotes the acceleration of a flame to form the initial shock front. Good design practice should minimize the number of components producing turbulence and the intensity of turbulence they produce. However, the experimental observation of the quenching of flames, on account of flame stretching at high levels of turbulence, makes it impossible to give definitive advice on this aspect. There may be scope for considering the possibility of safety measures, based on high levels of turbulence. Evidently, further work is required in this area before firm recommendations could be made.

Finally, the importance of more mundane matters such as good housekeeping and regular inspection, testing and maintenance cannot be over-emphasized. Together with the choice of optimum operating procedures, these produce a crucial contribution to the safety of plant.

There is some information available on the effects of a difference between the velocity of the axial stress wave in containment walls and that of the detonation itself [362, 363]. However, there have been no systematic studies of the relationship between the axial and hoop stress waves and the properties of the detonation. The following section concerns the requirements for a fuller understanding of this relationship. It is based on the concept that it may be possible to contemplate designing parts of an installation to withstand the effects of a detonation. For instance, when the sole protection consists of a detonation trap, it is necessary to ensure safe containment upstream of it. Again, in a complex chemical process plant, there may be wide variations in the operating pressures of the various sections, and containment may be feasible in the regions of lower pressure.

Economic considerations dictate the inclusion of items of standard design, such as pumps and compressors, in plant at potential risk from the effects of a detonation. In certain instances, it may be possible to confer some degree of protection by designing an outer shell with a planned degree of expansion, when it is subjected to the effects of an internal explosion. A further example of the possible use of planned deformation is lightweight ducting, from which it is planned that at all times fuel is absent, used solely to transport air to a particular processing vessel. It is obviously necessary to ensure that the deformation is below that at which cracking commences. Furthermore, it is necessary to be able to estimate the effects of any previous explosion on the deformation produced by a subsequent one, in order to decide whether the replacement of slightly distorted components is necessary. Some of the questions raised by these issues are examined in Section 9.3.

A more general approach to design of plant at risk is concerned with minimizing both the amplitude of local peaks in pressure, resulting from the ignition of the precompressed medium, and the areas over which they can occur. This philosophy could well be combined with strengthening of components at particular risk. Whilst the theoretical aspects of mitigating peak pressures have been discussed in Chapter 6, Section 9.4 emphasizes the practical aspects and considers areas in which further work is required.

The final section deals with a number of miscellaneous areas in which further work could result in a more secure foundation of some of the proposed safety measurements. In particular, it concentrates on the problems associated with quantifying the properties of fronts with a spacing of transverse waves approximately that of the characteristic dimensions of the containment.

9.2 Stress waves in confining walls

There have been no systematic studies of the influence of the properties of detonation waves and those of the wall itself on the stress wave propagating therein. This is explicable in terms of the problems associated with effects of end walls, of transmission across joints and of the possible interactions of reflected longitudinal stress waves with the circumferential wave. However, there are a number of general points to be made. For instance, the velocity of the longitudinal elastic waves, v_e, in most metals is considerably higher than the C–J velocity in most media at temperatures likely to be normally encountered in processing plant. Indeed, at normal temperatures, only the C–J velocity in fuel-rich mixtures of hydrogen and oxygen approaches v_e. At the maximum operating temperatures likely to be encountered in plant, the C–J velocity may be doubled. However, as v_e is proportional to $\sqrt{(E/\rho)}$, where E is the Young's modulus and ρ the density of the wall material, it is virtually independent of temperature. Even at high temperatures v_e will generally exceed D_{CJ}, and the walls downstream of the initiation of a detonation first experience the effects of the stress wave.

An interesting exception is the case of lead for which $\nu_e = 1.2\,\text{km s}^{-1}$. Many of Dixon's [19, 162] classical studies of detonations were conducted in a long pipeline of lead, wound in a spiral around a drum. Typical detonation velocities in the experimental mixtures used were $2.0 \leq D_{CJ} \leq 2.5\,\text{km s}^{-1}$, resulting in a typical delay of about 0.1 s between the arrival of the detonation wave and the stress wave at the end of the tube. However, there is no mention in his publications of anomalous effects attributable to this unusual set of conditions.

On account of the more normal delay between the prior arrival of the elastic wave and the detonation itself, separate treatments of their effects on the extension at a given position appear justifiable. Experimental studies of longitudinal elastic waves in metal walls of detonation tubes [362, 363] suggest that initial elastic strains are <0.2% and can be neglected in comparison with those due to the arrival of the detonation itself. However, the scant available data suggest that this is not true of hoop strains which should be taken into account in calculating the final plastic strain.

A number of fundamental features of elastic deformation deserve investigation. By analogy with the effects of compressible boundary layers in reducing detonation velocities and in possible quenching effects, significant circumferential deformations ahead of the detonation front might be expected to moderate its velocity. This feature might repay examination in thin-walled tubes. Furthermore, the effects of wide variations in local pressure (as for instance occur with galloping waves) in modulating the stress waves have not been studied. There are serious experimental difficulties in monitoring the elastic strains produced by detonations in marginally-detonable media. It would be valuable to confirm the common assumption that the effects of the precursor elastic waves on permanent deformations are negligible.

9.3 Planned deformations as safety measures

Some of the situations in which consideration might be given to allowing a safe degree of deformation to result from a detonation have been discussed in Section 9.1. However, as will become apparent, it would be wise to confine any application to regions in which flame acceleration rather than a steady detonation is likely. In such regions the problems in predicting the behaviour of the structure are somewhat reduced by the finite rates of rise in pressure prior to the formation of a shock, and the lower pressures involved.

In the aftermath of an explosion, it will be necessary to replace any deformed components in order to guarantee their performance in any subsequent explosion. Consequently, an appropriate design criterion might be based on extensions to just below that at which cracks are initiated. Little is known about the relationship between the extent of yield and the generation of cracks in structures subjected to a detonation. It will be recalled that experiments with detonations in stoichiometric gas mixtures, producing C–J pressures well in excess of those at which failure of the structure was expected to occur, resulted in cracking commencing well before the maximum extension occurred [364]. Only when the C–J pressure was approximately that at which flat plates and thin beams might be expected to fail did the full extension of the structure precede cracking. Evidently this finding needs to be confirmed for the much less uniform pressures produced by detonations in marginal mixtures, before it could be promulgated as a general design criterion. Further uncertainties exist, in terms of the effects of variations in the material properties of the wall (brought about for instance by welds, differences in heat treatment, corrosion, etc.) on the relationship between deformation and cracking. In the absence of information on these aspects, it would be necessary to incorporate very wide factors of safety in planning deformations resulting from detonation waves.

In the absence of such information, planned deformations are only likely to be applied as a last resort. However, there are more positive aspects to the requirement for information on the relationship between yield and cracking, produced by detonation pressures. One concerns the dangers associated with fragments acting as shrapnel in the event of a detonation. It is evidently crucial that the inlet sections of detonation traps are designed to be crackproof. Furthermore, such information relating yield and cracking would be of great value in the investigation of explosions in plant.

9.4 Designing to minimize the effects of local peaks in pressure

There are two principal mechanisms whereby pressures arise exceeding those predicted by simple unidimensional theories of detonations. The first of these involves the interactions of compression waves produced during the initiation of the front. An example of this is pressure-piling or cascading. It will be recalled that this involves a steady front propagating through a medium compressed by the earlier phase of flame acceleration. The pressure ratio across the front, corresponding approximately with the C–J value, is enhanced by the pre-compression ratio. In this instance, it involves the end distant from initiation being closed. A closed end in the intiation section can also result in anomalously high pressures. These occur when a retonation wave reflected from the initiation end overtakes and coalesces with the incident front to produce an overdriven detonation. Both effects can result in high pressures existing over an extended length of pipeline. However, apart from avoiding the inclusion of closed ends, there is little scope for designing to mitigate these effects.

The other mechanism applies to established fronts, and, with the possible exception of galloping waves, results in highly localized regions of high pressure. It involves the ignition of the medium compressed by the precursor front behind its associated transverse fronts. As such it applies to both confined and freely expanding detonations. However, its effects are enhanced in waves in marginally-detonable media and by interactions with changes in confinement. In the latter case, the weakening of the precursor front at expansive surfaces increases the distances involved in explosive reinitiation, resulting in an extension of the distances over which abnormally high pressures extend.

In practice detonations are highly unlikely to occur in anything other than a marginally-detonable medium, so that ameliorative techniques are confined to the design of changes in confinement, which should be gradual. More precisely, the characteristic distance over which they occur should be at least comparable with, and preferably greater than, the change in characteristic dimension of the surrounding walls. For instance, expansions and contractions in cross-section should be in the form of nozzles with smoothly curved walls, rather than in the form of truncated cones. This allows for a gradual change in strength of the wave at the walls and the requisite distance for an averaging process to occur in its strengthening at the inlet to a contraction and the outlet of an expansion. In addition, the resultant decrease in non-planarity of the front appears to promote a smoother re-establishment process, minimizing the amplitude of peak pressures and the distance over which they are generated.

Sharp elbow-like bends should be avoided. Ideally, they should be sweeping with a ratio of radius of curvature to radius of the bore of five or more [296, 320, 321]. This contributes to preserving the planarity of the front as it propagates around the bend. Similar considerations apply to junctions. It is particularly important to allow sufficient distance between the inlet and the outer dividing wall for attenuation of the complete periphery of the front, before it suffers normal reflection there.

In addition to applying these design concepts, it may be necessary to contemplate local strengthening of contractions in area and surfaces which may experience normal reflection. It is important to ensure that such reinforcement extends some diameters downstream, in order to allow sufficient distance for the expansion fronts to attenuate the complete periphery of the wave. Although the exit of an expansion nozzle is a compressive surface, it is presented with a weakened front, so that its strengthening need not be so extensive.

Finally, the suggested design concepts may have an additional advantage in that they may well be less effective as generators of turbulence, and consequently reduce the acceleration of a flame in the early stages of an incipient detonation.

9.5 Suggestions for further studies of detonations

The primary yardstick used in listing suggestions for further work is their potential value in securing the foundations on which safety recommendations have been based. Although there is a clear need to identify unambiguous ways of discriminating between the effects of a fully-developed detonation from those of an accelerating flame–shock complex, these are only likely to result from more speculative studies. It appears to be logical to follow the outline of the text in listing areas in which further work is required.

In this context, further work based on unidimensional concepts is evidently of little value. Whilst an empirical appreciation of the effects of the properties of the detonable medium and of its confinement on the structure of fronts has emerged, there remain a number of important questions. For instance, how general a phenomenon are galloping fronts? Are the ratios of peak to C–J pressures, observed in the limited number of media tested, common to all media in which such waves can occur? There is need for further experimental work on galloping waves, both in a wider range of gaseous mixtures of fuel and oxidant, and more particularly in self-decomposing media, suspensions of flammable dusts and flammable aerosols. Presently, it is possible to indicate approximately the limiting local pressure profiles produced by detonations in mixtures of fuel and oxidant, in the absence of changes in confinement. However, further studies, aimed at a more accurate estimate of the maximum variation possible in pressure profile of detonations in premixed gases, would be desirable for designs based on the response of the surrounding walls. The situation in respect to detonations in thermally unstable fuels, dust clouds and fogs is even less satisfactory, there being no direct experimental evidence on the maximum possible variation in pressure history.

The problems in categorizing what media are detonable under what conditions of composition, pressure, temperature and confinement have been dealt with in some detail. The obvious definition of such a medium, as one suitably conditioned to produce natural transverse waves, is not helpful, in the absence of a complete understanding of their origin in the presence and the absence of surrounding walls. Furthermore, the application of a theoretical analysis of the nature of transverse waves to a medium of unknown explosive potential would require a detailed knowledge of the chemical kinetics of the processes governing the release of chemical energy. These are not likely to be available in the near future for the less common fuels and oxidants, mixtures of which may be capable of supporting a detonation. Consequently, assessment of detonability, on the basis of flammability tests and detonation experiments, carried out under confinement and over a limited range of critical pressures, temperatures and possibly compositions, is likely to continue for the foreseeable future. In this context, the most urgent problem concerns the development of methods of extrapolating from known limits of detonability in confined mixtures to limits for unconfined media. Some clues to the appropriate approach might be obtained from a definitive answer to the question of whether partly confined or freely expanding detonations are possible in self-decomposing gases, aerosols and dust clouds. Such work on the latter two media should also serve to fill in gaps in our knowledge of an area in which information is singularly sparse.

There are a number of industrial situations in which hybrid mixtures of flammable dust particles or of oil droplets with flammable gases or vapours and oxidant can be formed. There are grave difficulties in deciding on the detonability of such media, when the concentration of flammable gas or vapour is below the fuel-lean limit. Examples are the air space above a partly oil-filled crankcase in which a mixture of oil droplets, oil vapour and air occurs. In mine galleries there may well be a concentration of methane below the lower limit of flammability, together with a readily available supply of coal dust on the walls, floor and roof of the gallery. The problem in deciding on the detonability of such media is compounded by the variety of ways in which they can be produced in and around processing plant. Examples are the flash evaporation into air of a compressed fuel of low boiling point and the formation of dust clouds by the scouring action of the flow of the unburnt mixture ahead of a flame on a deposit of combustible dust. It is likely that both flammability and detonability limits of these hybrid mixtures vary with the size distribution of particles or droplets, and (in the case of particles) their shapes, volatile contents and rates of release, so that considerable experimental effort will be required to determine limits.

Another interesting problem is the prediction of limits for clouds of particles in air of explosives such as TNT, containing insufficient oxygen for their stoichiometric decomposition. In the absence of air, the detonation of individual particles of the condensed explosive will result in individual blast fronts which eventually coalesce in a pipeline to produce a planar front, or in unconfined situations, a spherical wave. In air, it is possible to conceive the greater potential release of energy, as the particles produce a stoichiometric mixture of products, resulting in the transition to a detonation wave. On account of the number of industrial situations in which hybrid mixtures can be produced and our lack of knowledge of their properties, their study merits high priority.

From the standpoint of the control and prevention of detonations, the interest in further work on the various processes of initiation is, in confined media, essentially academic. Given the presence of a potentially detonable gaseous mixture, it is necessary to consider the consequences of a detonation, since it is virtually impossible to guarantee the exclusion of ignition sources of sufficient energy to produce an initial flame. There is possibly an argument for work on initiation in confined dust clouds and aerosols, for which initiation energies are considerably higher. There is greater promise in studies of the possible effect of the composition of two-phase systems on the critical energies of initiation of unconfined detonations.

Many of the recommendations for further work on the structure of detonation waves apply to detonations interacting with changes in confinement. Of particular importance, in terms of interaction with structures, are more detailed examinations of fronts with widely spaced transverse waves. In addition to identifying the range of amplitudes in local pressure, the studies should identify the distances over which anomalously high pressures persist. In this context, further studies are needed of waves in marginally-detonable media interacting with inert and compressible boundary layers, to confirm their quenching effect. Similarly, further work with marginal detonations is required on their refraction at an interface and their propagation through gradients in composition. Available information is mainly for nearly planar waves [307, 338, 339], and its analysis based on concepts of planarity. There are indications that anomalous results may be produced by non-planar fronts [339]. Finally, there is evidence that reaction zones in two-phase detonations are thicker and occur further behind the transverse waves than in homogeneous media. Thus there is a need for data on the modifications to pressure profiles produced by such waves during their interactions with changes in confinement.

The importance of a comparison of damage produced by the nearly planar detonation waves with that resulting from the non-planar fronts in marginally-detonable media has already been discussed. It is also worth emphasizing that to date there have been no measurements of combined hoop and axial stresses produced by a detonation travelling through a tube. However, there must be some questions on how best to utilize the results of further studies of the damage produced by detonations. These concern the probable variations in the materials of construction of a plant, brought about by differences in residual stresses, in heat treatments and the presence of welded sections etc. The benefits from such work are likely to accrue principally in terms of investigations of damage caused by explosions.

There are a number of features of the control and prevention of detonations which merit further attention. For instance, economic benefits would be derived from more precise estimates of the minimum concentration of inhibitor and of the distance over which it must be dispersed. The accurate determination of dispersal distances is particularly important in the case of dust clouds. For instance, it is possible to conceive of the inhibitor quenching chemical reaction zones without significantly cooling the particles. In the disturbed flow, resulting from the injection of the inhibitor, the velocities of the still-hot particles and that of the inhibitor-containing gas will be different. The movement of the particles into regions in which the inhibitor is absent could well result in the re-establishment of the detonation. Thus there is a justifiable tendency to specify excessive additions of the relatively expensive quenching agents.

It is always difficult to ensure that the length of a detonation tube downstream of any change in cross-section is sufficient for the re-establishment of a front of uniform velocity. Consequently, testing of further designs of quenching and suppression devices must be carried out with great care. In particular, any test which results in a pressure wave propagating through the outlet of the device should be verified. It will be recalled that the shock wave–flame complex can propagate for long distances in the case of galloping waves, and that run-up distances, for the formation of a detonation from an accelerating flame, are even greater.

References

It may be helpful to list particularly fruitful sources of information on detonation waves in gaseous media. The Combustion Institute, Pittsburgh, Pennsylvania, organize biennial symposia, abbreviated in the following to *Nth Symp. (Int.) Comb.*, a complete session of which is generally devoted to papers on gaseous detonations. In addition, the Combustion Institute's journal, 'Combustion and Flame' (*Comb. and Flame*) publishes a wide selection of papers on detonations. The equivalent Soviet publication is *Combustion, Explosion and Shock Waves*.

Two more somewhat amorphous organizations hold biennial meetings in which a wide selection of contributions on detonations are presented. The first of these has organized a series of International Colloquia on Gasdynamics of Explosions and Reactive System (ICOGERS). The papers from these meetings have appeared in a number of different media, including *Acta Astronautica* (published by Pergamon Press) and *Progress in Astronautics and Aeronautics* (published by the American Institute of Astronautics and Aeronautics, AIAA). The second informal group organizes international symposia on research on shock waves. Latterly, papers at these meetings have been published under the auspices of a committee in the host country under the title 'Shock Tubes and Waves', *The Proceedings of the Nth International Symposium on Shock Tubes and Waves*.

There have been a series of meetings held under the auspices of the Institute of Chemical Engineers (UK) (Inst. Chem. Eng. in references) or those of the European Federation of Chemical Engineering on 'Loss Prevention and Safety Promotion in the Process Industries' following on from earlier meetings under the title 'Symposia on Chemical Process Hazards' which contain a selection of papers on gaseous detonations. Again, the American Institute of Chemical Engineers (abbreviated to A.I.Ch.E. in references) has arranged a number of symposia under the general title of 'Loss Prevention', in the proceedings of which a number of valuable contributions on aspects of gaseous detonation waves have appeared. One note of caution may be appropriate in drawing attention to the fact that the series of symposia published under the general title 'Nth International Symposium on Detonation' deal almost exclusively with condensed explosives.

A number of journals in the list of references are no longer extant. Thus, *Archiwum Procesow Spalania* (*Arch. Proc. Span.*) has been replaced by *Archivum Combustionis* (*Arch. Comb.*). The *Journal of the American Rocket Society* (*ARSJ*) has effectively been taken over by the *Journal of the American Institute of Aeronautics and Astronautics* (*AIAAJ*).

The abbreviation USBM is used for United States Bureau of Mines, AERE for Atomic Energy Research Establishment, Comb. Inst. for the Combustion Institute and NACA for the National Advisory Committee for Aeronautics (now NASA). OSRD is the Office of Scientific Research Development (defunct from 1947). The *Journal of Hazardous Materials* has been abbreviated to *J. Haz. Mat.* and *Discussions of the Faraday Society* as *Dis. Far. Soc.* The journal *Fire Prevention Science and Technology* published by the Fire Prevention Association (UK) is denoted as *Fire Prev. Sci. and Tech.*, *Progress in Aerospace Sciences* as *Prog. Aero. Sci.* and *Progress in Energy and Combustion Sciences* as *Prog. Energy Comb. Sci.* The remaining abbreviations used are standard ones and should be readily recognizable.

In order to give a clue to the nature of the contents of each reference, the title of the contribution is given. It is hoped that this will prove to be particularly useful in cases in which the reference covers a much wider field than the particular aspect quoted. The titles themselves appear with a capital letter for each word where the article is in a unique publication rather than in a periodical.

1. Gugan, K. (1979) *Unconfined Vapour Cloud Explosions*, Inst. Chem. Eng., Rugby, UK.
2. Nettleton, M. A. (1976) Some aspects of vapour cloud explosion, *J. Occ. Acc.*, **1**, 149.
3. Zel'dovich, Ya. B. and Kompaneets, A. S. (1960) *Theory of Detonation*, Academic Press, New York.
4. Shchelkin, K. J. and Troshin, Ya. K. (1965) *Gas Dynamics of Combustion*, Mono Book Corporation, Baltimore.
5. Soloukhin, R. I. (1966) *Shock Waves and Detonations in Gases*, Mono Book Corporation, Baltimore.
6. Gruschka, H. D. and Wecken, F. (1971) *Gasdynamic Theory of Detonation*, Gordon and Breach, New York.
7. Fickett, W. and Davis, W. C. (1979) *Detonation*, University of California Press, Berkeley.
8. Lewis, B. and Von Elbe, G. (1961) *Combustion, Flames and Explosions of Gases*, Academic Press, New York.
9. Strehlow, R. A. (1968) *Fundamentals of Combustion*, International Textbook Corporation, Scranton, USA.
10. Bradley, J. N. (1962) *Shock Waves in Chemistry and Physics*, Chapman and Hall,

London.
11. Gaydon, A. G. and Hurle, I. R. (1963) *The Shock Tube in High Temperature Chemical Physics*, Chapman and Hall, London.
12. Stull, D. R. (1977) Fundamentals of fire and explosion, *A.I.Ch.E. Monograph Series No. 10*, **73**, A.I.Ch.E., New York.
13. Bodurtha, F. T. (1980) *Industrial Explosion Prevention and Control*, McGraw-Hill, New York.
14. Voitsekhovskii, B. V., Mitrofanov, V. V. and Topchian, M. E. (1963) 'Structure of a Detonation Front in Gases', *Izd-vo Sibirsk, Odtel.* Adak. Nauk SSR, Novosibirsk, Translation 1966, Wright-Patterson Air Force Base Report, FTD-MT-64-527 (AD-633-821).
15. Strehlow, R. A. (1968) Gas phase detonations: recent developments, *Comb. and Flame*, **12**, 81.
16. Edwards, D. H. (1969) A survey of recent work on the structure of detonation waves, *12th Symp. (Int.) Comb.*, Comb. Inst., Pittsburgh.
17. Lee, J. H. and Moen, I. O. (1980) The mechanism of transition from deflagration to detonation in vapour cloud explosions, *Prog. Energy Comb. Sci.*, **6**, 359.
18. Munday, G. (1971) Detonations in vessels and pipelines, *Chem. Eng.*, **248**, 135.
19. Dixon, H. B. (1903) On the movements of the flame in the explosion of gases, *Phil. Trans. Roy. Soc.*, **200**, 315.
20. Chapman, D. L. (1899) On the rate of explosions in gases, *Phil. Mag.*, **47**, 90.
21. Jouguet, E. (1905) Sur la propagation des reactions chimiques dans les gaz, *J. Maths. Pure Appl.*, **7**, 347.
22. Zel'dovich, Ya. B. (1940) On the theory of the propagation of detonation in gaseous systems, *J. Exp. Theor. Phys. USSR*, **10**, 524. Translation NACA Tech. Memo 1261.
23. von Neumann, J. (1942) Progress report on the theory of detonation waves, OSRD Rept. No. 549.
24. Doring, W. (1943) Uber den detonationsvorgang in gasen, *Ann. Physik*, **43**, 421.
25. Fay, J. A. (1959) Two-dimensional gaseous detonations: velocity deficit, *Phys. Fluids*, **2**, 283.
26. Tsuge, S. (1971) The effects of boundaries on the velocity deficit and the limits of gaseous detonations, *Comb. Sci. and Tech.*, **3**, 195.
27. Campbell, C. and Woodhead, D. W. (1927) Striated photographic records of explosion waves, *J. Chem. Soc.*, 1572.
28. Campbell, C. and Finch, A. C. (1928) Striated photographic records of explosion waves. II. An explanation of the striae, *J. Chem. Soc.*, 2094.
29. Bird, P. F., Duff, R. E. and Schott, G. L. (1964) Hug, A Fortranfap code for computing normal shock and detonation wave parameters in gases, *Los Alamos Scientific Laboratory Report* LA 2980.
30. Mader, C. L. (1967) Fortran Sin, a one-dimensional hydrodynamic code for problems which include chemical reactions, elastic-plastic flow, spalling and phase transitions, *Los Alamos Scientific Laboratory Report* LA 3720 UC-32.
31. Gordon, S. and McBride, B. J. (1971) Computer program for calculation of complex equilibrium compositions, NASA SP-273 (internal report).
32. Soloukhin, R. I. (1966) Multiheaded structure of gaseous detonation, *Comb. and Flame*, **10**, 51.
33. Edwards, D. H., Walker, J. R. and Nettleton, M. A. (1984) On the propagation of detonation waves along wedges, *Arch. Comb.*, **4**, 197.

34. Brochet, C. and Sayous, M. (1981) Detection Method for the Deflagration to Detonation Transition in Gaseous Explosive Mixtures, 'Gasdynamics of Detonations and Explosions' (eds J. R. Bowen, N. Manson, A. K. Oppenheim and R. I. Soloukhin) *Prog. Astro. Aero*, **75**, 73.

35. Edwards, D. H., Thomas, G. O. and Nettleton, M. A. (1979) The diffraction of a planar detonation wave at an abrupt change in area, *J. Fluid Mech.*, **95**, 79.

36. Edwards, D. H. and Lawrence, T. R. (1965) Ionisation measurements in detonation waves, *Proc. Roy. Soc.*, **286**, 415.

37. Barreto, E., Reynolds, S. I. and Jurenka, H. (1974) Ignition of hydrocarbons and the thermalisation of electrical discharges, *J. App. Phys.*, **45**, 3317.

38. Edwards, D. H., Fearnley, P. J. and Nettleton, M. A. (1984) Detonation limits of clouds of coal dust in mixtures of oxygen and nitrogen, *1st Int. Coll. Explosibility Industrial Dusts*, Polish Academy of Science, Warsaw, p. 168.

39. White, D. R. (1957) On the existence of higher than normal detonation pressures, *J. Fluid Mech.*, **2**, 513.

40. Ginsburgh, I. (1958) Abnormaly high detonation pressures in a shock tube, *J. App. Phys.*, **29**, 1381.

41. Duff, R. E., Knight, H. T. and Wright, H. R. (1954) Some detonation properties of acetylene gas, *J. Chem. Phys.*, **22**, 1618.

42. Nettleton, M. A. and Young, D. M. (1973) The propagation of flames in gases in large diameter pipes, *Comb. Inst. Europ. Symp.* (ed. F. J. Weinberg), Academic Press, New York.

43. Hellen, T. K. (1980) BERSAFE, *Berkeley Structural Analysis by Finite Elements*, CEGB, Berkeley Nuclear Laboratories, UK.

44. Hellen, T. K. (1982) A Description of the BERSAFE System. In *Finite Element Systems: A Handbook*, (ed. C. A. Brebbia), Springer-Verlag, New York.

45. Laffitte, P. and Bouchet, R. (1959) Suppression of explosion waves in gaseous mixtures by means of fine powders, *7th Symp. (Int.) Comb.*, Butterworths, London, p. 504.

46. Anon (1946) German techniques for handling acetylene in chemical operations, *FIAT Final Report*, HMSO, London, p. 720.

47. Cubbage, P. (1963) The Protection by Flame Traps of Pipelines Containing Combustible Mixtures, *2nd Symp. Chem. Proc. Hazards*, Inst. Chem. Eng., London, p. 29.

48. Flessner, M. F. and Bjorklund, R. A. (1981) Control of Gas Detonations in Pipelines, *A.I.Ch.E. 14th Loss Prev. Symp.*, A.I.Ch.E., New York, p. 113.

49. Nettleton, M. A. (1976) Alleviation of blast waves from large vapour clouds, *J. Occ. Acc.*, **1**, 3.

50. Gaydon, A. G. and Wolfhard, H. G. (1953) *Flames, Their Structure, Radiation and Temperature*, Chapman and Hall, London, p. 293.

51. Taylor, G. I. (1950) The dynamics of the combustion products behind plane and spherical detonation fronts in explosives, *Proc. Roy. Soc.*, **A200**, 235.

52. Lewis, B. and Friauf, J. B. (1930) Explosions in detonating gas mixtures. I. Calculation of rates of explosions in mixtures of hydrogen and oxygen and the influence of rare gases, *J. Am. Chem. Soc.*, **52**, 3905.

53. Berets, D. G., Greene, E. F. and Kistiakowsky, G. B. (1950) Gaseous detonations. I. Stationary waves in hydrogen–oxygen mixtures, *J. Am. Chem. Soc.*, **72**, 1080.

54. Edwards, D. H., Williams, G. T. and Breeze, J. C. (1959) Pressure and velocity measurements on detonation waves in hydrogen–oxygen mixtures, *J. Fluid Mech.*, **6**, 497.

55. Strehlow, R. A. and Crooker, A. J. (1974) The structure of marginal detonation waves, *Acta Astronaut.*, **1**, 303.

56. Gordon, W. E. (1949) Pressure Measurement in Gaseous Detonation by Means of Piezoelectric Gauges, *3rd Symp.* (*Int.*) *Comb.*, Williams and Wilkins, Baltimore, p. 579.

57. Brochet, G., Manson, N., Rouze, M. and Struck, W. (1963) Influence de la pression initiale sur la celerité des détonations stables dans les melanges stoechiometriques propane–oxygene et ethylene–oxygene, *Compt. Rendu Hebd. Sceances Acad. Sci.*, **257**, 2412.

58. Duff, R. E., Knight, H. T. and Rink, J. P. (1958) Precision flash X-ray determination of density ratio in gaseous detonations, *Phys. Fluids*, **1**, 393.

59. White, D. R. (1961) Turbulent structure of gaseous detonation, *Phys. Fluids*, **4**, 465.

60. Fay, J. A. and Opel, G. (1958) Two-dimensional effects in gaseous detonation waves, *J. Chem. Phys.*, **29**, 955.

61. Edwards, D. H., Jones, T. G. and Price, B. (1963) Observations on oblique shock waves in gaseous detonations, *J. Fluid Mech*, **17**, 21.

62. Wagner, H. Gg. (1962) Recherches experimentales sur la structure de la zone de reaction dans les détonations de gaz, *Colloque Int. du CNRS*, No. 109, 235 (Paris).

63. Price, R. B. (1963) *An Investigation of Detonation Waves in Hydrogen–Oxygen Mixtures*, Ph.D. Thesis, Department of Physics, University College of Wales, Aberystwyth.

64. Voitsekhovskii, B. V., Mitrofanov, V. V. and Topchian, M. E. (1969) Investigation of the Structure of Detonation Waves in Gases, *12th Symp.* (*Int.*) *Comb.*, Comb. Inst., Pittsburgh, p. 829.

65. Strehlow, R. A., Liaugminas, R., Watson, R. H. and Eyman, J. R. (1967) Transverse Wave Structures in Detonations, *11th Symp.* (*Int.*) *Comb.*, Comb. Inst., Pittsburgh, p. 683.

66. Strehlow, R. A., Maurer, R. E. and Rajan, S. (1970) Transverse waves in detonations. I. Spacing in the hydrogen–oxygen system, *AIAAJ*, **7**, 323.

67. Strehlow, R. A. and Engel, C. D. (1970) Transverse waves in detonations. II. Structure and spacing in H_2-O_2, $C_2H_2-O_2$, $C_2H_4-O_2$ and CH_4-O_2 systems, *AIAAJ*, **7**, 492.

68. Campbell, C. and Woodhead, W. (1926) The ignition of gases by an explosion wave. I. Carbon monoxide and hydrogen mixtures, *J. Chem. Soc.*, 3010.

69. Bone, W. A. and Fraser, R. P. (1929) A photographic investigation of flame movements in carbonic oxide–oxygen explosions, *Phil. Trans. Roy. Soc.*, **A228**, 197.

70. Bone, W. A. and Fraser, R. P. (1931) A photographic investigation of flame movements in gaseous explosions. VI. The phenomenon of spin in detonations, *Phil. Trans. Roy. Soc.*, **A230**, 373.

71. Bone, W. A., Fraser, R. P. and Wheeler, W. H. (1936) A photographic investigation of flame movements in gaseous explosions. VII. The phenomenon of spin in detonation, *Phil. Trans. Roy. Soc.*, **A235**, 29.

72. Manson, N. (1946) Sur la structure des ondes explosives dites helicoidales dans les mélanges gazeux, *Compt. Rendu Acad. Sci.*, **222**, 46.

73. Fay, J. A. (1952) A mechanical theory of spinning detonation, *J. Chem. Phys.*, **20**, 942.

74. Predvoditelev, A. J. (1959) Concerning Spin Detonation, *7th Symp.* (*Int.*) *Comb.*, Butterworths, London, p. 760.

75. Martin, F. J. and White, D. R. (1959) The Formation and Structure of Gaseous Detonation Waves, *7th Symp.* (*Int.*) *Comb.*, Butterworths, London, p. 856.

76. Duff, R. E. (1961) Investigation of spinning detonation and detonation stability, *Phys. Fluids*, **4**, 1427.

77. Schott, G. L. (1965) Observations of the structure of spinning detonation waves, *Phys. Fluids*, **8**, 850.

78. Jones, H. (1976) The dynamics of spinning detonations, *Proc. Roy. Soc.*, **A348**, 299.

79. Gordon, W. E., Mooradian, A. J. and Harper, S. A. (1959) Limit and Spin Effects in Hydrogen–Oxygen Detonations, *7th Symp.* (*Int.*) *Comb.*, Butterworths, London, p. 752.

80. Barthel, H. O. (1974) Predicted spacings in hydrogen–oxygen–argon detonations, *Phys. Fluids*, **17**, 1547.

81. Munday, G., Ubbelohde, A. R. and Wood, I. F. (1968) Fluctuating detonation in gases, *Proc. Roy. Soc.*, **A306**, 171.

82. Mitrofanov, V. V., Subbotin, V. A. and Topchian, M. E. (1963) On measurements of pressure in a transverse spinning wave, *Zh. prikl. Mekh., i Tekh. Fiz.*, **3**, 45.

83. Schultz-Grunow, F. (1978) The mechanism of spinning detonations, *Int. J. Heat and Mass Trans.*, **21**, 63.

84. Manson, N., Brochet, C., Brossard, J. and Pujol, Y. (1963) Vibratory Phenomena and Instability of Self Sustained Detonations in Gases, *9th Symp.* (*Int.*) *Comb.*, Academic Press, New York, p. 461.

85. St Cloud, J. C., Guerraud, C., Brochet, C. and Manson, N. (1972) Quelques particularites des detonations très instables dans les melanges gazeux, *Acta Astronautica*, **17**, 487.

86. Edwards, D. H. and Morgan, J. M. (1977) Instabilities in detonation waves near the limits of propagation, *J. Phys. D*, **10**, 2377.

87. Urtiew, P. A. and Oppenheim, A. K. (1966) Experimental observations of the transition to detonation in an explosive gas, *Proc. Roy. Soc.*, **A295**, 13.

88. Strehlow, R. A. (1970) Multidimensional detonation wave structure, *Acta Astronautica*, **15**, 345.

89. Edwards, D. H., Thomas, G. O. and Nettleton, M. A. (1981) Diffraction of a Planar Detonation Wave in Various Fuel-Oxygen Mixtures at an Area Change, 'Gasdynamics of Detonations and Explosions', (eds J. R. Bowen, W. Mason, A. K. Oppenheim and R. I. Soloukhin) *Prog. Astro. Aero.*, **75**, 341.

90. Lundstrom, E. A. and Oppenheim, A. K. (1969) On the influence of non-steadiness on the thickness of detonation waves, *Proc. Roy. Soc.*, **A310**, 759.

91. Liaugminas, R., Barthel, H. O. and Strehlow, R. A. (1973) Mach stem structure in exothermic systems, *Comb. and Flame*, **20**, 19.

92. Takai, R., Yoneda, R. and Hikita, T. (1975) Study of Detonation Wave Structure, *15th Symp.* (*Int.*) *Comb.*, Comb. Inst., Pittsburgh, p. 69.

93. Duff, R. E. and Finger, M. (1965) Stability of a spherical detonation wave, *Phys. Fluids*, **8**, 764.

94. Tarver, C. M. (1982) Chemical energy release in the cellular structure of gaseous detonation waves, *Comb. and Flame*, **46**, 135.

95. Strehlow, R. A. and Biller, J. R. (1969) On the strength of transverse waves in gaseous detonations, *Comb. and Flame*, **13**, 577.

96. Vasiliev, A. A., Gavrilenco, T. P. and Topchian, M. E. (1972) On the Chapman–Jouguet surface in multi-headed gaseous detonations, *Acta Astronautica*, **17**, 499.

97. Edwards, D. H., Jones, A. T. and Phillips, D. E. (1976) The location of the Chapman–Jouguet surface in a multiheaded detonation wave, *J. Phys. D*, **9**, 1331.

98. Bull, D. C., Elsworth, J. E., Shuff, P. J. and Metcalfe, E. (1982) Detonation cell structures in fuel/air mixtures, *Comb. and Flame*, **45**, 7.

99. Moen, I. O., Murray, S. B., Bjerketvedt, D., Rinnan, A., Knystautas, R. and Lee, J. H. (1983) Diffraction of Detonation from Tubes into a Large Fuel–Air Explosive Cloud, *19th Symp. (Int.) Comb.*, Comb. Inst., Pittsburgh, p. 635.

100. Westbrook, C. K. (1982) Chemical kinetics of hydrocarbon oxidation in gaseous detonations, *Comb. and Flame*, **46**, 191.

101. Bull, D. C. (1979) Concentration limits to the initiation of unconfined detonation in fuel–air mixtures, *Trans. Inst. Chem. Eng.*, **57**, 219.

102. Atkinson, R., Bull, D. C. and Shuff, P. J. (1980) Initiation of spherical detonation in hydrogen/air, *Comb. and Flame*, **39**, 287.

103. Westbrook, C. K. and Urtiew, P. A. (1983) Chemical Kinetic Prediction of Critical Parameters in Gaseous Detonations, *19th Symp. (Int.) Comb.*, Comb. Inst., Pittsburgh, p. 615.

104. Tarver, C. M. (1982) Chemical energy release in one-dimensional detonation waves in gaseous explosives, *Comb. and Flame*, **46**, 111.

105. Nettleton, M. A. (1974) Influence of preflame reactions on combustion of hydrocarbons in shock-heated air, *Fuel*, **53**, 99.

106. Erpenbeck. J. J. (1963) Structure and Stability of the Square Wave Detonation, *9th Symp. (Int.) Comb.*, Academic Press, New York, p. 442.

107. Erpenbeck, J. J. (1964) Stability of idealised one-dimensional detonations, *Phys. Fluids*, **7**, 684.

108. Erpenbeck, J. J. (1965) Stability of idealised one-reaction detonations of zero activation energy, *Phys. Fluids*, **8**, 1192.

109. Erpenbeck, J. J. (1966) Detonation stability for disturbances of small transverse wavelength, *Phys. Fluids*, **9**, 1293.

110. Barthel, H. O. (1972) On reaction zone–shock front coupling in detonations, *Phys. Fluids*, **15**, 43.

111. Chiu, K. W. and Lee, J. H. (1976) A simplified version of the Barthel model for transverse wave spacings in gaseous detonations, *Comb. and Flame*, **26**, 353.

112. Nettleton, M. A. (1984) The Transition from Deflagration to Detonation in Confined Gaseous Mixtures: Effects of Flame Structure, *Workshop on Gas Flame Structure*, USSR Academy of Sciences, Siberian Division, Novosibirsk, p. 98 (in Russian).

113. Michels, H. J., Munday, G. and Ubbelohde, A. R. (1970) Detonation limits in mixtures of oxygen and homologous hydrocarbons, *Proc. Roy. Soc.*, **A319**, 461.

226   *References*

114. Borisov, A. A., Kogarko, S. M. and Lyumbimov, A. V. (1968) Ignition of fuel films behind shock waves in air and oxygen, *Comb. and Flame*, **12**, 465.
115. Rae, D. (1971) Coal-dust explosions in large tubes. In *Shock Tube Research* (eds J. L. Stollery, A. G. Gaydon and P. R. Owen), Chapman and Hall, London, p. 47.
116. Brochet, C. (1966) *Contribution a l'etude des Detonations Instables dans les Melanges Gazeux*, Thesis, Faculty of Science, Poitiers University.
117. Strehlow, R. A. (1973) Unconfined Vapour Clouds – An Overview, *14th Symp. (Int.) Comb.*, Comb. Inst., Pittsburgh, p. 1189.
118. Zel'dovich, Ya. B., Kogarko, S. M. and Simonov, N. N. (1956) An experimental investigation of spherical detonations in gases, *Sov. Phys. Tech. Phys.*, **1**, 1689.
119. Bull, D. C., Elsworth, J. E., Hooper, G. and Quinn, C. P. (1976) A study of spherical detonation in mixtures of methane and oxygen diluted with nitrogen, *J. Phys. D.*, **9**, 1991.
120. Bull, D. C., Elsworth, J. E. and Hooper, G. (1978) Initiation of spherical detonations in hydrocarbon–air mixtures, *Acta Astronautica*, **5**, 997.
121. Kogarko, S. M., Adushkin, V. V. and Lyamin, A. C. (1966) An investigation of spherical detonations of gas mixtures, *Int. Chem. Eng.*, **6**, 393.
122. Knystautas, R. and Lee, J. H. (1976) On the effective energy for the direct initiation of gaseous detonations, *Comb. and Flame*, **27**, 221.
123. Matsui, H. and Lee, J. H. (1976) Influence of electrode geometry and spacing on the critical energy for direct initiation of spherical gaseous detonations, *Comb. and Flame*, **27**, 217.
124. Knystautas, R., Lee, J. H. and Guirao, C. M. (1982) The critical tube diameter for detonation failure in hydrocarbon–air mixtures, *Comb. and Flame*, **48**, 63.
125. Edwards, D. H., Hooper, G. and Morgan, J. M. (1976) An experimental investigation of spherical detonations, *Acta Astronautica*, **3**, 117.
126. Mitrofanov, V. V. and Soloukhin, R. I. (1965) The diffraction of multifront detonation waves, *Sov. Phys. Dokl.*, **9**, 1055.
127. Soloukhin, R. I. and Ragland, K. W. (1969) Ignition processes in expanding detonations, *Comb. and Flame*, **13**, 295.
128. Klimkin, V. F., Soloukhin, R. I. and Wolansky, P. (1973) Initial stages of a spherical detonation directly initiated by a laser spark, *Comb. and Flame*, **21**, 111.
129. Cassutt, L. H. (1961) Experimental investigation of unconfined detonations in gaseous H_2–O_2–N_2 mixtures, *ARSJ*, **31**, 1122.
130. Freiwald, H. and Koch, H. W. (1963) Spherical Detonations of Acetylene–Oxygen–Nitrogen Mixtures as a Function of Nature and Strength of Initiation, *9th Symp. (Int.) Comb.*, Academic Press, New York, p. 275.
131. Benedick, W. B., Kennedy, J. D. and Morosin, B. (1970) Detonation limits of unconfined hydrocarbon–air mixtures, *Comb. and Flame*, **15**, 83.
132. Benedick, W. B. (1979) High explosive initiation of methane–air detonations, *Comb. and Flame*, **35**, 89.
133. Moen, I. O., Donato, M., Knystautas, R. and Lee, J. H. (1981) The Influence of Confinement on the Propagation of Detonations near the Detonability Limits, *18th Symp. (Int.) Comb.*, Comb. Inst., Pittsburgh, p. 1615.
134. Bretherick, L. (1979) *Handbook of Reactive Chemical Hazards*, Butterworths, London.

135. Miller, S. A. (1965) *Acetylene, its Properties, Manufacture and Uses*, Ernest Benn, London.
136. Miller, S. A. and Penny, E. (1960) Hazards in Handling Acetylene in Chemical Processes, Particularly under Pressure, *Symp. Chem. Proc. Hazards*, Inst. Chem. Eng., London, p. 87.
137. Penny, E. (1956) The velocity of detonation in compressed acetylene, *Disc. Far. Soc.*, No. 22, 156.
138. Mayes, H. A. (1956) (A comment on [137]) *Disc. Far. Soc.*, No. 22, 213.
139. Getzinger, R. W., Bowen, J. R., Oppenheim, A. K. and Boudart, M. (1965) Steady Detonations in Gaseous Ozone, *10th Symp. (Int.) Comb.*, Comb. Inst., Pittsburgh, p. 779.
140. Campbell, G. A. and Rutledge, P. V. (1972) Detonation of Hydrogen Peroxide Vapour, *Inst. Chem. Eng. Symp. Series No. 33*, Inst. Chem. Eng., London, p. 37.
141. Anon (1960) *Acetylene Transmission for Chemical Synthesis*, International Acetylene Association, New York.
142. Paillard, C., Dupre, G. and Combourieu, J. (1973) Etude de la detonation de composes endothermiques gaseux. I. Celerités de detonation de l'azoture de chlore dans des tubes cylindriques. Limites de detonation de l'azoture de chlore et de l'azoture d'hydrogene, *J. Chem. Phys.*, 70, 811.
143. Paillard, C., Dupre, G., Lisbet, R., Combourieu, J., Fokeev, V. P. and Gvozdeva, L. G. (1979) A study of hydrogen azide detonation with heat transfer at the wall, *Acta Astronautica*, 6, 227.
144. Paillard, C., Dupre, G. and Combourieu, J. (1974) Etude de la detonation de composés endothermiques gazeux. II. Propagation et conditions critiques d'extinction dans des tubes capillaires de la flamme de decomposition de l'azoture de chlore gaseux pur ou dilué, *J. Chem. Phys.*, 71, 175.
145. Dupre, G., Paillard, C. and Combourieu, J. (1971) Chaleur de decomposition et limites d'inflammabilitie de l'azoture de brome, *Compt. Rendu Acad. Sci.*, 273, 445.
146. Laffitte, P., Combourieu, J., Hajal, J., Ben-Caid, M. and Moreau, R. (1967) Characteristics of Chlorine Dioxide Decomposition Flames at Reduced Pressures, *11th Symp. (Int.) Comb.*, Comb. Inst., Pittsburgh, p. 941.
147. Ribovich, J., Murphy, J. and Watson, R. (1975/1977) Detonation studies with nitric oxide, nitrous oxide, nitrogen tetroxide, carbon monoxide and ethylene, *J. Haz. Mat.*, 1, 275.
148. Steacie, E. W. R. (1931) The thermal decomposition of diazomethane, *J. Phys. Chem.*, 35, 1493.
149. Courtney, W. G., Clark, W. J. and Slough, C. M. (1962) Ignition of ethylene oxide vapour, *ARSJ*, 32, 1530.
150. Bajpai, S. N. (1980) Flammability of ethylene oxide in steriliser operations, *Loss Prevention*, 13, 119, A.I.Ch.E., New York.
151. Pesetsky, B., Cawse, J. N. and Wyn, W. T. (1980) Liquid phase decomposition of ethylene oxide, *Loss Prevention*, 13, 123, A.I.Ch.E., New York.
152. Pesetsky, B. and Best, R. D. (1980) Methane requirements for ethylene oxide handling and storage, *Loss Prevention*, 13, 132, A.I.Ch.E., New York.
153. Griffiths, J. F. and Perche, A. (1981) The Spontaneous Decomposition, Oxidation and Ignition of Ethylene Oxide under Rapid Compression, *18th Symp. (Int.) Comb.*, Comb. Inst., Pittsburgh, p. 893.

154. Jarvis, H. C. (1971) Butadiene explosion at Texas City – 1, *Loss Prevention*, **5**, 57, A.I.Ch.E., New York.

155. Freeman, R. H. and McCready, M. P. (1971) Butadiene explosion at Texas City – 2, *Loss Prevention*, **5**, 61, A.I.Ch.E., New York.

156. Keister, R. G., Pesetsky, B. I. and Clark, S. W. (1971) Butadiene explosion at Texas City – 3, *Loss Prevention*, **5**, 67, A.I.Ch.E., New York.

157. Kinney, C. R. and Slysh, R. S. (1960) On the Mechanism of Carbonisation of Benzene, Acetylene and Diacetylene at 1200 °C, *Proc. 4th Conf. Carbon*, Pergamon Press, Oxford, p. 301.

158. Hou, K. C. and Anderson, R. C. (1963) Comparative studies of pyrolysis of acetylene, vinylacetylene and diacetylene, *J. Phys. Chem.*, **67**, 1579.

159. Zabetakis, M. G. (1965) Flammability characteristics of combustible gases and vapours, *USBM Bull 627*.

160. Breton, J. (1936) *Recherches sur la Detonation des Melanges Gazeux*, Theses Faculte des Sciences, Univ. Nancy.

161. Craven, A. D. and Greig, T. R. (1968) The development of detonation over-pressures in pipelines, *J. Chem. E. Symp. Series* No. **25**, 41, Inst. Chem. Eng., London.

162. Dixon, H. B. (1893) The rate of explosion in gases, *Phil. Trans. Roy. Soc.*, **A184**, 97.

163. Munday, G., Ubbelohde, A. R. and Wood, I. F. (1968) Marginal detonation in cyanogen–oxygen mixtures, *Proc. Roy. Soc.*, **A306**, 179.

164. Kistiakowsky, G. B., Knight, H. T. and Malin, M. E. (1952) Gaseous detonations. III. Dissociation energies of nitrogen and carbon monoxide, *J. Chem. Phys.*, **20**, 876.

165. Miles, J. E. P., Munday, G. and Ubbelohde, A. R. (1966) Condensation effects in the detonation of tetramethyl silane, *Proc. Roy. Soc.*, **A291**, 167.

166. Carlson, G. A. (1973) Spherical detonations in gas–oxygen mixtures, *Comb. and Flame*, **21**, 383.

167. Nettleton, M. A. (1980) Detonation and flammability limits of gases in confined and unconfined situations, *Fire Prev. Sci. and Tech*. No. **23**, 29.

168. Nettleton, M. A. (1980) Comments on 'Concentration Limits to the Initiation of Unconfined Detonation in Fuel–Air Mixtures' (D. C. Bull), *Trans. J. Chem. E.*, **58**, 281.

169. Sokolik, A. S. and Shchelkin, K. I. (1934) Detonation in gaseous mixtures, *J. Phys. Chem (USSR)*, **5**, 1459.

170. Lee, J. H., Knystautas, R., Guirao, C., Bekesy, A. and Sabbagh, S. (1972) On the instability of H_2–Cl_2 detonations, *Comb. and Flame*, **18**, 321.

171. Levin, V. A., Chernyi, G. G., Teodorczyk, A., Wolanski, P. and Wojcicki, S. (1978) The initiation of a detonation process in H_2–Cl_2 mixture, *Arch. Term. Span.*, **9**, 613.

172. Bollinger, L. E., Laughrey, J. A. and Edse, R. (1962) Experimental detonation velocities and induction distances in hydrogen–nitrous oxide mixture, *ARSJ*, **32**, 81.

173. Coward, H. F. and Jones, G. W. (1952) Limits of flammability of gases and vapours, *USBM Bull. 503*.

174. Sargent, H. B. (1957) How to design a hazard-free system, *Chem. Eng.*, **64**, 250.

175. Nettleton, M. A. (1960) *Some Aspects of the Pyrolysis of Acetylene*, PhD Thesis, University of London.

176. Gray, P. and Waddington, T. C. (1956) Thermochemistry and reactivity of oxides. I. Thermochemistry of the inorganic oxides, *Proc. Roy. Soc.*, **A235**, 106.
177. Bollinger, L. E., Fong, M. C. and Edse, R. (1961) Experimental measurements and theoretical analysis of detonation induction distance, *ARSJ*, **31**, 588.
178. Miles, J. E. P., Munday, G. and Ubbelohde, A. R. (1962) Effects of additives on marginal detonations in gases, *Proc. Roy. Soc.*, **A269**, 165.
179. Munday, G., Ubbelohde, A. R. and Wood, I. F. (1968) Dual detonation regimes in hydrogen–oxygen and deuterium–oxygen mixtures, *Proc. Roy. Soc.*, **A306**, 159.
180. Munday, G., Ubbelohde, A. R. and Wood, I. F. (1968) Mass effects in detonation limits, *Proc. Roy. Soc.*, **A303**, 397.
181. Rae, D. and Thompson, W. (1979) Experiments on prevention and suppression of coal-dust explosions by bromochlorodifluoromethane and prevention by carbon tetrachloride, *Comb. and Flame*, **35**, 131.
182. Nettleton, M. A. and Stirling, R. (1974) The influence of additives on the burning of clouds of coal particles in shocked gases, *Comb. and Flame*, **22**, 407.
183. Jones, G. W., Kennedy, R. E. and Spolan, I. (1948) Effects of hydrocarbons and other gases on the explosibility of acetylene, *USBM Report 4196*.
184. Burgoyne, J. H. and Cohen, L. (1954) The effect of drop size on flame propagation in liquid aerosols, *Proc. Roy. Soc.*, **A225**, 375.
185. Bull, D. C., McLeod, M. A. and Mizner, G. A. (1981) Detonation of unconfined fuel aerosols, 'Gasdynamics of Detonations and Explosions' (eds J. R. Bowen, N. Manson, A. K. Oppenheim and R. I. Soloukhin), *Prog. Astro. and Aero.*, **75**, 61.
186. Cramer, F. B. (1963) The Onset of Detonation in a Droplet Combustion Field, *9th Symp. (Int.) Comb.*, Academic Press, New York, p. 482.
187. Nicholls, J. A., Dabora, E. K. and Ragland, K. W. (1966) A study of heterogeneous detonations, *Acta Astronautica*, **12**, 9.
188. Ragland, K. W., Nicholls, J. A. and Dabora, E. K. (1968) Observed structure of spray detonations, *Phys. Fluids*, **11**, 2377.
189. Nicholls, J. A., Dabora, E. K. and Ragland, K. W. (1969) Drop-size Effects in Spray Detonations, *12th Symp. (Int.) Comb.*, Comb. Inst., Pittsburgh, p. 19.
190. Bowen, J. R., Ragland, K. W., Steffes, F. J. and Loflin, T. C. (1971) Heterogeneous Detonations Supported by Fuel Fogs as Films, *13th Symp. (Int.) Comb.*, Comb. Inst., Pittsburgh, p. 1131.
191. Ragland, K. W. and Garcia, C. F. (1972) Ignition delay measurements in two-phase detonations, *Comb. and Flame*, **18**, 53.
192. Pierce, T. H. and Nicholls, J. A. (1973) Time Variation in the Reaction Zone Structure of Two-phase Spray Detonations, *14th Symp. (Int.) Comb.*, Comb. Inst., Pittsburgh, p. 1277.
193. Fry, R. S. and Nicholls, J. A. (1974) Blast initiation and propagation of cylindrical detonations in MAPP–air mixtures, *AIAAJ*, **12**, 1703.
194. Bar-or, R., Sichel, M. and Nicholls, J. A. (1981) The Propagation of Cylindrical Detonations in Monodisperse Sprays, *18th Symp. (Int.) Comb.*, Comb. Inst., Pittsburgh, p. 1599.
195. Fry, R. S. and Nicholls, J. A. (1975) Blastwave initiation of Gaseous and Heterogeneous Cylindrical Detonation Waves, *15th Symp. (Int.) Comb.*, Comb. Inst., Pittsburgh, p. 43.
196. Nettleton, M. A. (1977) Shock-wave chemistry in dusty gases and fogs, a review, *Comb. and Flame*, **28**, 3.

197. Strauss, W. A. (1968) Investigation of the detonation of aluminium powder–oxygen mixtures, *AIAAJ*, **6**, 1753.

198. Tulis, A. J. (1980) On the Detonation of Unconfined Aluminium Particles Dispersed in Air, 'Shock Tubes and Waves', *Proc. 12th Int. Symp. Shock Tubes and Waves* (eds A. Lifshitz and J. Rom), Magnes Press, Jerusalem.

199. Tulis, A. J. and Selman, R. (1983) Detonation Tube Studies of the Aluminium Particles, *19th Symp. (Int.) Comb.*, Comb. Inst., Pittsburgh, p. 655.

200. Nettleton, M. A. and Stirling, R. (1973) Detonations in suspensions of coal dust in oxygen, *Comb. and Flame*, **21**, 307.

201. Kauffman, C. W. and Nicholls, J. A. (1982) Dust explosion research at University of Michigan 'Fuel–Air Explosions', *Proc. Int. Conf. on Fuel–Air Explosions*, University of Waterloo Press, Canada, p. 623.

202. Kimber, G. M. and Gray, M. D. (1967) Rapid devolatilisation of small coal particles, *Comb. and Flame*, **11**, 360.

203. Zalesinski, M. (1980) Private Communication.

204. Wolanski, P. (1981) Problems of Dust Explosions, *1st Spec. Meet. (Int.) Comb. Inst.*, French Section, Comb. Inst., Paris, p. 497.

205. Lesnyak, S. A. and Slutskii, V. G. (1977) Theory of propagation limits of heterogeneous (gas-film) detonation, *Comb. Explos. and Shock Waves*, **13**, 626.

206. Terao, K. (1977) Explosion limits of hydrogen–oxygen mixture as a stochastic phenomenon, *Jap. J. App. Phys.*, **16**, 29.

207. Terao, K., and Sawada, R. (1979) Stochastic aspect of the transition to detonation, *Jap. J. App. Phys.*, **18**, 1463.

208. Fay, J. A. (1953) Some Experiments on the Initiation of Detonation in $2H_2 + O_2$ Mixtures by Uniform Shock Waves, *4th Symp. (Int.) Comb.*, Williams and Wilkins, Baltimore, p. 501.

209. Steinberg, M. and Kaskan, W. (1955) The Ignition of Combustible Mixtures by Shock Waves, *5th Symp. (Int.) Comb.*, Reinhold Publishing Corporation, New York, p. 664.

210. Strehlow, R. A. and Cohen, A. (1960) Shock-initiated detonations, *Phys. Fluids*, **3**, 319.

211. Strehlow, R. A. and Cohen, A. (1962) Initiation of detonation, *Phys. Fluids*, **5**, 97.

212. Strehlow, R. A. and Dyner, H. B. (1963) One-dimensional detonation initiation, *AIAAJ*, **1**, 591.

213. Gilbert, R. B. and Strehlow, R. A. (1966) Theory of detonation initiation behind reflected shock waves, *AIAAJ*, **4**, 1777.

214. Kling, R. and Maman, A. (1961) Detonation in Shock-Wave Ignited Kerosene-Air Mixture, *8th Symp. (Int.) Comb.*, Williams and Wilkins, Baltimore, p. 1096.

215. Zaitsev, S. G. and Soloukhin, R. I. (1962) Study of Combustion of an Adiabatically-heated Gas Mixture, *8th Symp. (Int.) Comb.*, Williams and Wilkins, Baltimore, p. 344.

216. Soloukhin, R. I. (1964) On detonation in gases preheated with shock waves, *Zh. Prikl. Mekhan. i Tekhn. Fiz.*, **4**, 42.

217. Soloukhin, R. I. (1964) Detonation waves in gases, *Sov. Phys. Usp.*, **6**, 523.

218. Edwards, D. H., Thomas, G. O. and Williams, T. L. (1981) Initiation of detonation by steady planar incident shock waves, *Comb. and Flame*, **43**, 187.

219. Zaitsev, S. G. and Soloukhin, R. I. (1958) Combustion in an adiabatically heated

gaseous mixture, *Proc. USSR Acad. Sci. Phys. Chem.*, **122**, 745.

220. Oran, E. S. and Kailasanath, K. (1983) Ignition of flamelets behind incident shock waves and the transition to detonation, *NRL Report* **5030**, Naval Research Laboratory, Washington DC.

221. Bradley, J. N., Capey, W. D. and Farajii, F. (1980) The Effect of Reaction Exothermicity on Shock Propagation, 'Shock Tubes and Waves', *Proc. 12th Int. Symp. on Shock Tubes and Waves* (eds A. Lifshitz and J. Rom), Magnes Press, Jerusalem.

222. Urtiew, P. A. and Oppenheim, A. K. (1968) Transverse flame–shock interactions in an explosive gas, *Proc. Roy. Soc.*, **A304**, 379.

223. Inomata, T. and Suzuki, M. (1977) The transition from deflagration in ethylene–oxygen systems, *Bull. Chem. Soc. Jap.*, **50**, 2247.

224. Wojcicki, S. and Zalesinski, M. (1973) The Mechanism of Transition from Combustion to Detonation in a Mixture of Coal Dust and Gaseous Oxidiser, 'Recent Developments in Shock Tube Research', *Proc. 9th Int. Shock Tube Symp.* (eds D. Bershader and W. Griffith), Stanford University Press, p. 821.

225. Zalesinki, M. and Wojcicki, S. (1981) Generation of Detonations by Two-stage Burning, 'Gasdynamics of Detonations and Explosions' (eds J. R. Bowen, N. Manson, A. K. Oppenheim and R. I. Soloukhin), *Prog. Astro. Aero.*, **75**, 439.

226. Zalesinki, M., Kusmierz, A., Teodorczyk, A. and Wojcicki, S. (1981) The Models of Transition from Combustion in a Coal Dust and Oxygen Mixture, *1st Spec. Meet. (Int.), Comb. Inst.*, French Section, Comb. Inst., Paris, p. 503.

227. Oran, E. S., Boris, J. P., Young, T. R., Fritts, M. J., Picone, M. J. and Fyfe, D. (1982) Numerical simulations of fuel–air explosions: current methods and capabilities, 'Fuel–Air Explosions', *Proc. Int. Conf. on Fuel–Air Explosions*, University of Waterloo Press, Canada, p. 447.

228. Hasson, A., Avinor, M. and Burcat, A. (1983) Transition from deflagration to detonation, spark ignition and detonation characteristics of ethylene–oxygen mixtures in a tube, *Comb. and Flame*, **49**, 13.

229. Lee, J. H., Knystautas, R. and Guirao, C. M. (1975) Critical Power Density for Direct Initiation of Unconfined Gaseous Detonations, *15th Symp. (Int.) Comb.*, Comb. Inst., Pittsburgh, p. 53.

230. Nettleton, M. A. (1975) Explosions due to faults in electrical equipment, *Elec. Rev.*, **197**, 116.

231. Nettleton, M. A. (1984) The generation of blast-waves from confined electrical discharges, *IEE Proc.*, **131**, 96.

232. Carlson, G. A. (1971) Generation of maximum shock wave pressures by exploding wires, *J. App. Phys.*, **42**, 2155.

233. Strachan, D. B. (1979) Categorising exploding-wires for use in detonation studies, *Comb. and Flame*, **36**, 305.

234. Zalesinski, M., Kalbarczyk, M. and Wojcicki, S. (1973) Investigation into the explosion mechanism of coal dust with gaseous oxidiser, *Arch. Proc. Span.*, **4**, 199.

235. Daiber, J. W. and Thompson, H. M. (1967) Laser-driven detonation waves in gases, *Phys. Fluids*, **10**, 1162.

236. Lee, J. H. and Knystautas, R. (1969) Laser spark ignition of chemically reactive gases, *AIAAJ*, **7**, 312.

237. Benedick, W. B. (1982) Review of large scale fuel–air explosion tests and tech-

niques, 'Fuel–Air Explosions', *Proc. Int. Conf. on Fuel–Air Explosions*, University of Waterloo Press, Canada, p. 507.

238. Hikita, T. (1975) *Experimental Results of Explosions and Fires of Liquid Ethylene Facilities*, Safety Information Centre, Institution for Safety of High Pressure Gas Engineering, Tokyo.

239. Kirk-Othmer (1980) *Encyclopedia of Chemical Technology*, **9**, John Wiley and Sons, London.

240. Baker, W. E. (1973) *Explosions in Air*, University of Texas Press, London.

241. Funk, J. W., Murray, S. B., Ward, S. and Moen, I. O. (1982) A brief description of the DRES fuel–air explosives testing facility and current research program, 'Fuel–Air Explosions', *Proc. Int. Conf. on Fuel–Air Explosions*, University of Waterloo Press, Canada, 565.

242. Manson, N. and Ferrie, F. (1953) Contribution to Study of Spherical Detonation Waves, *4th Symp. (Int.), Comb.*, Williams and Wilkins, Baltimore, p. 486.

243. Desbordes, D. (1973) *Celerite de Propagation des Detonations Spheriques Divergentes dans les Melanges Gazeux*, Theses di 3ème Cycle, Poitiers.

244. Lee, J. H. and Ramamurthi, K. (1976) On the concept of the critical size of a detonation kernel, *Comb. and Flame*, **27**, 331.

245. Edwards, D. H., Hooper, G., Morgan, J. M. and Thomas, G. O. (1978) The quasisteady regime in critically-initiated detonation waves, *J. Phys. D*, **11**, 2103.

246. Kekez, M. M. and Savic, P. (1974) A hypersonic interpretation of the development of the spark channel in gases, *J. Phys. D*, **7**, 620.

247. Kekez, M. M. and Savic, P. (1980) Subnanosecond schlieren study of the spark channel tip: part 1, *6th Int. Conf. Gas Discharges*, IEE, London, p. 221.

248. Gerber, N. and Bartos, J. M. (1974) Strong spherical blast waves in a dust-laden gas, *AIAAJ*, **12**, 120.

249. Sichel, M. (1977) A simple analysis of the blast initiation of detonations, *Acta Astronautica*, **4**, 409.

250. Burgess, D. S. and Zabetakis, M. G. (1973) Detonation of a Flammable Cloud Following a Propane Pipeline Break, *USBM Report. Investigation 7752*.

251. Clancey, V. J. (1975) The Phenomenology of Vapour Explosions in Free Space, *2nd Europ. Symp. Comb.*, French Section, Comb. Inst., Paris, p. 238.

252. Strehlow, R. A., Luckritz, R. T., Adamczyk, A. A. and Shimpi, S. A. (1979) The blast wave generated by spherical flames, *Comb. and Flame*, **35**, 297.

253. Moore, S. R. and Weinberg, F. J. (1981) High propagation rates of explosions in large volumes of gaseous mixtures, *Nature*, **290** (5801), 39.

254. Moore, S. R. and Weinberg, F. J. (1981) On the Role of Radiation in the Propagation of Unconfined Vapour Cloud Explosions, *1st Spec. Meeting (Int.) Comb. Inst.*, French Section, Comb. Inst., Paris, p. 301.

255. Moore, S. R. and Weinberg, F. J. (1983) A study of the role of radiative ignition in the propagation of large explosions, *Proc. Roy. Soc.*, **A385**, 373.

256. Bray, K. N. C., Libby, P. A., Masuya, G. and Moss, J. B. (1981) Turbulence production in premixed turbulent flames, *Comb. Sci. and Tech.*, **25**, 127.

257. Bray, K. N. C. and Moss, J. B. (1981) Spontaneous Acceleration of Unconfined Flames, *1st Spec. Meeting (Int.) Comb. Inst.*, French Section, Comb. Inst., Paris, p. 7.

258. Urtiew, P. A. and Tarver, C. M. (1981) Effects of the cellular structure on the behaviour of gaseous detonation waves in transient conditions, 'Gasdynamics of

Detonations and Explosions' (eds J. R. Bowen, N. Manson, A. K. Oppenheim and R. I. Soloukhin) *Prog. Astr. and Aero.*, **75**, 370.

259. Matsui, H. and Lee, J. H. (1979) On the Measure of the Relative Detonation Hazards of Gaseous Fuel–Oxygen and Air Mixtures, *17th Symp. (Int.) Comb.*, Comb. Inst., Pittsburgh, p. 1269.

260. Ballal, D. R. and Lefebvre, A. H. (1975) The Influence of Flow Parameters on Minimum Ignition Energy and Quenching Distance, *15th Symp. (Int.) Comb.*, Comb. Inst., Pittsburgh, p. 1473.

261. Ballal, D. R. and Lefebvre, A. H. (1977) Ignition and flame quenching in flowing gaseous mixtures, *Proc. Roy. Soc.*, **A357**, 163.

262. Ballal, D. R. and Lefebvre, A. H. (1978) Ignition and flame quenching of quiescent fuel mists, *Proc. Roy. Soc.*, **A364**, 277.

263. Ballal, D. R. and Lefebvre, A. H. (1979) Ignition and flame quenching of flowing heterogeneous fuel–air mixtures, *Comb. and Flame*, **35**, 155.

264. Ballal, D. R. and Lefebvre, A. H. (1981) A General Model of Spark Ignition for Gaseous and Liquid Fuel-Air Mixtures, *18th Symp. (Int.) Comb.*, Comb. Inst., Pittsburgh, p. 1737.

265. Ballal, D. R. (1983) Further studies on the ignition and flame quenching of quiescent dust clouds, *Proc. Roy. Soc.*, **A385**, 1.

266. Rose, H. E. and Priede, T. (1959) Ignition Phenomena in Hydrogen–Air Mixtures, *7th Symp. (Int.) Comb.*, Butterworths, London, p. 436.

267. Rose, H. E. and Priede, T. (1959) An Investigation of the Characteristics of Spark Discharges as Employed in Ignition Experiments, *7th Symp. (Int.) Comb.*, Butterworths, London, p. 454.

268. Abdel-Gayed, R. G. and Bradley, D. (1981) A two-eddy theory of premixed turbulent flame propagation, *Phil. Trans. Roy. Soc.*, **A301**, 1.

269. Jahn, G. (1934) *Der Zundvorgang in Gasgemischen*, Oldenbourg, Berlin.

270. Ballal, D. R. (1983) Flame propagation through dust clouds of carbon, coal, aluminium and magnesium in an environment of zero gravity, *Proc. Roy. Soc.*, **A385**, 21.

271. Andrews, G. E. and Bradley, D. (1972) Determination of burning velocities: a critical review, *Comb. and Flame*, **18,** 133.

272. Nettleton, M. A. and Stirling, R. (1967) The ignition of clouds of particles in shock-heated oxygen, *Proc. Roy. Soc.*, **A300**, 62.

273. Nettleton, M. A. and Stirling, R. (1971) The combustion of clouds of coal particles in shock-heated mixtures of oxygen and nitrogen, *Proc. Roy. Soc.*, **A322**, 207.

274. Bollinger, L. E. (1964) Experimental detonation velocities and induction distances in hydrogen–air mixtures, *AIAAJ*, **2**, 131.

275. Steen, H. and Schampel, K. (1983) Experimental Investigations on the Run-up Distance of Gaseous Detonations in Large Pipes, *4th Int. Symp. Loss Prevention and Safety Promotion Process Industries*, **III**, E23, Inst. Chem. Eng., Rugby.

276. Nettleton, M. A. (1973) Flame Acceleration in Particulate Suspensions – a Method of Assessing the Vulnerability of Pipelines, *Comb. Inst. Europ. Symp.*, Academic Press, New York, p. 372.

277. Jones, H. (1958) Accelerated flames and detonations in gases, *Proc. Roy. Soc.*, **A248**, 333.

278. Nettleton, M. A. (1975) Shock-waves in dust/droplet suspensions with particular

234   References

reference to the initiation of a detonation, *Arch. Term. Span.*, **6**, 457.

279. Pawel, D., van Tiggelen, P. J., Vasatko, H. and Wagner, H. Gg. (1970) Initiation of detonation in various gas mixtures, *Comb. and Flame*, **15**, 173.

280. Ginsburgh, I. and Bulkley, W. L. (1963) Hydrocarbon–air detonations: industrial aspects, *Chem. Eng. Prog.*, **59**, 82.

281. Jost, W. (1946) *Explosion and Combustion Processes in Gases*, McGraw-Hill, New York (Quoting unpublished work by Lafitte and Dumanois)

282. Laffitte, P. (1928) Influence of temperature on the formation of explosive waves, *Compt. Rendu*, **186**, 951.

283. Baumann, W., Urtiew, P. A. and Oppenheim, A. K. (1961) On the influence of tube diameter on the development of gaseous detonation, *Zeitschrift fur Elektrochemie*, **65**, 895.

284. Laffitte, P. (1923) On the formation of an explosive wave, *Compt. Rend.*, **176**, 1392.

285. Hattwig, M. (1980) Detonationanlaufstreecken von Gasgemeschen in Rohren großen Durchmessers, *Amts. Mitteilungsblatt der Budenstalt fur Materialprufung (BAM)*, **10**, 274.

286. Bartknecht, W. (1971) *Brenngas und Staubexplosionen Forschungsbericht*, F49 der Bundesinstitut fur Arbeitsschutz.

287. Glass, I. I. and Hall, J. G. (1959) *Handbook of Supersonic Aerodynamics, Sect. 18, Shock Tubes*, Bureau of Naval Weapons, Washington, DC.

288. Egerton, A. and Gates, S. F. (1927) On detonation of acetylene and of pentane, *Proc. Roy. Soc.*, **A114**, 137.

289. Moen, I. O., Donato, M., Knystautas, R. and Lee, J. H. (1980) Flame acceleration due to turbulence produced by obstacles, *Comb. and Flame*, **39**, 21.

290. Moen, I. O., Donato, M., Knystautas, R. and Lee, J. H. (1981) Turbulent flame propagation and acceleration in the presence of obstacles, 'Gasdynamics of Detonations and Explosions' (eds J. R. Bowen, N. Manson, A. K. Oppenheim and R. I. Soloukhin), *Prog. Astro. and Aero.*, **75**, 33.

291. Chan, C., Moen, I. O. and Lee, J. H. (1983) Influence of confinement on flame acceleration due to repeated obstacles, *Comb. and Flame*, **49**, 27.

292. Fitt, J. S. (1981) Pressure piling: a problem for the process engineer, *Chem. Eng.* No. **368**, 237.

293. Heinrich, H-J. (1974) Zum ablaufgasexplosionen in mit rohrleitungen verbundenen behaltern, *BAM Berichte No. 28*, Der Budenstalt fur Materialprufung.

294. Sloan, S. A. and Nettleton, M. A. (1975) A model for the axial decay of a shock wave in a large and abrupt area change, *J. Fluid Mech.*, **71**, 769.

295. Sloan, S. A. and Nettleton, M. A. (1978) A model for the decay of a wall shock in a large abrupt area change, *J. Fluid Mech.*, **88**, 259.

296. Edwards, D. H., Thomas, G. O. and Nettleton, M. A. (1983) The diffraction of detonation waves in channels with 90° bends, *Arch. Comb.*, **3**, 65.

297. Bazhenova, T. V., Gvozdeva, L. G. and Nettleton, M. A. (1984) Unsteady interactions of shock waves, *Prog. Aero. Sci.*, **21**, 249.

298. Chester, W. (1954) The quasi-cylindrical shock tube, *Phil. Mag.*, **45**, 1293.

299. Chisnell, R. F. (1957) The motion of a shock wave in a channel with applications to cylindrical and spherical shock waves, *J. Fluid Mech.*, **2**, 286.

300. Whitham, G. B. (1974) *Linear and Non-Linear Waves*, Wiley Interscience, London.

301. Liepman, H. W. and Roshko, A. (1957) *Elements of Gas Dynamics*, John Wiley and Sons, New York.
302. Libouton, J-C., Dormal, M. and van Tiggelen, P. J. (1981) Reinitiation processes at the end of the detonation cell, 'Gasdynamics of Detonations and Explosions' (eds J. R. Bowen, N. Manson, A. K. Oppenheim and R. I. Soloukhin), *Prog. Astro. and Aero.*, **75**, 358.
303. Bazhenova, T. V., Gvozdeva, L. G., Lobastov, Ya.S., Naboko, I. M., Nemkov, R. G. and Predvoditeleva, O. A. (1968) *Shock Waves in Real Gases*, Nauka Press, Moscow, Translation NASA TT F-585.
304. Gvozdeva, L. G., Bazhenova, T. V., Predvoditeleva, O. A. and Fokeev, V. P. (1969) Mach reflection of shock waves in real gases, *Acta Astronautica*, **14**, 503.
305. White, D. R. and Cary, K. H. (1963) Structure of gaseous detonation. II. Generation of laminar detonation, *Phys. Fluids*, **6**, 749.
306. Lee, J. H., Knystautas, R. and Lee, B. H. K. (1965) Structure of gaseous detonations in a convergent-divergent channel, *AIAAJ*, **3**, 1786.
307. Strehlow, R. A., Adamczyk, A. A. and Stiles, R. J. (1972) Transient studies of detonation waves, *Acta Astronautica*, **17**, 509.
308. Lee, J-H. and Glass, I. I. (1983) Pseudo-stationary oblique-shock-wave reflections in frozen and equilibrium air, *Prog. Aero. Sci.*, **21**, 33.
309. Jones, T. G. and Vlases, G. C. (1967) Pressure probes for research in plasma dynamics and detonation, *Rev. Sci. Instr.*, **38**, 1038.
310. Walker, J. R. (1983) *Confined Flame Propagation and Detonation Reflection*, Ph.D. Thesis, Department of Physics, University College of Wales, Aberystwyth.
311. Brabbs, T. A., Zlatarich, S. A. and Belles, F. E. (1960) Limitations of the reflected shock technique for studying fast chemical reactions, *J. Chem. Phys.*, **33**, 307.
312. Baum, F. A., Staniukovich, K. P. and Shekliter, B. I. (1959) *Physics of Explosions*, GIFML, Moscow.
313. Staniukovich, K. P. (1960) *Unsteady Motion of Continuous Media*, Pergamon Press, Oxford.
314. Gvozdeva, L. G. (1964) *Physical Gasdynamics*, USSR Academy of Sciences, Moscow.
315. Denisov, Yv. N. (1965) Wall collision of waves from one-dimensional gas detonations with large and negligibly small ignition and induction periods, *J. App. Mech. Tech. Phys.*, **2**, 64.
316. Makomaski, A. H. (1967) Normal reflection of a plane gaseous detonation wave in a tube, *NRC Mech. Eng. Dept. Rept. MT-58*.
317. Dremin, A. N. and Trofimov, V. S. (1965) On the Nature of the Critical Diameter, *10th Symp. (Int.) Comb.*, Comb. Inst., Pittsburgh, p. 893.
318. Shchelkin, K. I. (1959) Two cases of unstable combustion, *Sov. Phys. JETP*, **9**, 416.
319. Hide, R. and Millar, W. (1956) A Preliminary Investigation of Shocks in a Curved Channel, AERE, GP/R 1918.
320. Edwards, D. H., Fearnley, P. and Nettleton, M. A. (1983) Shock diffraction in channels with 90° bends, *J. Fluid Mech.*, **132**, 257.
321. Fearnley, P. and Nettleton, M. A. (1983) Pressures Generated by Blast Waves in Channels with 90° Bends, *4th Int. Symp. Loss Prevention and Safety Promotion*

Process Industries, **3**, E34, Inst. Chem. Eng., Rugby.

322. Dadone, A., Pandolfi, M. and Tamanini, F. 91971) Shock waves propagating in a straight duct with a side branch, 'Shock Tube Research' (eds J. L. Stollery, A. G. Gaydon and P. R. Owen), *Proc. 8th Int. Shock Tube Symp.*, Chapman and Hall, London, p. 17.

323. Sloan, S. A. and Nettleton, M. A. (1971) The propagation of weak shock waves through junctions, 'Shock Tube Research' (eds J. L. Stollery, A. G. Gaydon and P. R. Owen), *Proc. 8th Int. Shock Tube Symp.*, Chapman and Hall, London, p. 18.

324. Nettleton, M. A. (1973) Shock attenuation in a 'gradual' area expansion, *J. Fluid Mech.*, **60**, 209.

325. Edwards, D. H., Fearnley, P., Thomas, G. O. and Nettleton, M. A. (1981) Shocks and Detonations in Channels with 90° Bends, *1st Spec. Meeting (Int.) Comb. Inst.*, French Section, Comb. Inst., p. 431.

326. Ubbelohde, A. R. (1953) The Possibility of Weak Detonation Waves, *4th Symp. (Int.) Comb.*, Williams and Wilkins, Baltimore, p. 464.

327. Sommers, W. P., 1961, Gaseous detonation wave interactions with nonrigid boundaries, *ARSJ*, **31**, 1780.

328. Voitsekhovskii, B. V. (1959) Maintained detonations, *Sov. Phys. Dok.*, **4**, 1207 (Translated from *Dok. Acad. Nauk SSSR*, **129**, 1254).

329. Dabora, E. K., Nicholls, J. A. and Morrison, R. B. (1965) The Influence of a Compressible Boundary Layer on the Propagation of Gaseous Detonations, *10th Symp. (Int.) Comb.*, Comb. Inst., Pittsburgh, p. 817.

330. Adams, T. G. (1978) Do weak detonations exist? *AIAAJ*, **16**, 1035.

331. Williams, F. A. (1976) Quenching thickness for detonations, *Comb. and Flame*, **26**, 403.

332. Hinckley, W. M. and Yang, J. C. S. (1975) Analysis of rigid polyurethane foam as a shock mitigator, *Exper. Mech.*, **15**, 1.

333. Mooradian, A. J. and Gordon, W. E. (1951) Gaseous detonation. I. Initiation of detonation, *J. Chem. Phys.*, **19**, 1166.

334. Gvozdeva, L. G. (1961) The refraction of detonation waves incident on the boundary between two gas mixtures, *Sov. Phys. Tech. Phys.*, **6**, 527.

335. Jahn, R. G. (1956) The refraction of shock waves at a gaseous interface, *J. Fluid Mech.*, **1**, 457.

336. Paterson, S. (1948) The reflection of a plane shock wave at a gaseous interface, *Proc. Phys. Soc.*, **61**, 119.

337. Paterson, S. (1953) Contact Transmission of a Detonation, *4th Symp. (Int.) Comb.*, Williams and Wilkins, Baltimore, p. 468.

338. Donato, M., Donato, L. and Lee, J. H. (1981) Transmission of Detonations Through Composition Gradients, *1st Spec. Meeting (Int.) Comb. Inst.*, French Section, Comb. Inst., p. 467.

339. Sutton, P. (1985) *Detonation Wave Propagation in Inhomogeneous Media*, PhD Thesis, Department of Physics, University College of Wages, Aberystwyth.

340. Baker, W. E., Cox, P. A., Westine, P. S., Kulesz, J. J. and Strehlow, R. A. (1983) *Explosion Hazards and Evaluation*, Elsevier, Amsterdam.

341. Robinson, C. A. (1973) Special report: fuel air explosives, *Aviation Week and Space Technology*, 42.

342. Bazhenova, T. V., Fokeev, V. P., Lobastov, Yu., Brossard, J., Bonnet, T.,

Brion, B. and Charpentier, N. (1981) Influence of the nature of confinement on gaseous detonation, 'Gasdynamics of Detonations and Explosions' (eds J. R. Bowen, N. Manson, A. K. Oppenheim and R. I. Soloukhin), *Prog. Astro. and Aero.*, **75**, 87.

343. Smith, W. R. (1971) Shock produced strain relaxation in aluminium, 'Shock Tube Research' (eds J. L. Stollery, A. G. Gaydon and P. R. Owen), *Proc. 8th Int. Shock Tube Symp.*, Chapman and Hall, London, p. 59.

344. Tang, S. (1965) Dynamic response of a tube under moving pressure, ASCE, *J. Eng. Mech. Div.*, **91**, 97.

345. Andrews, E. H., Bernstein, L., Nurse, P. J. and Reed, P. E. (1971) Impact testing of plastics using a shock tube, 'Shock Tube Research' (eds J. L. Stollery, A. G. Gaydon and P. R. Owen), *Proc. 8th Int. Shock Tube Symp.*, Chapman and Hall, London, p. 60.

346. Cole, R. H. (1948) *Underwater Explosions*, Princeton University Press, Princeton.

347. Nettleton, M. A. (1979) Deformation of metallic components by explosive loads, *J. Occ. Acc.*, **2**, 99.

348. Dixon, H. B. and Cain, J. C. (1894) On the instantaneous pressures produced in the explosion wave, *Mem. Proc. Manchester Lit. and Phil. Soc.*, 174.

349. Jones, R. H. and Bower, J. (1898) On the instantaneous pressures produced on the collision of two explosive waves, *Manchester Memoirs*, **XLII**, 1.

350. Campbell, C., Littler, W. B. and Whitworth, C. (1932) The measurement of pressures developed in explosion waves, *Proc. Roy. Soc.*, **A137**, 380.

351. Payman, W. and Shepherd, W. C. F. (1936) Explosion waves and shock waves. IV. Quasi-detonation in mixtures of methane and air, *Proc. Roy. Soc.*, **A158**, 348.

352. Jacobs, R. B. (1959) Occurrence and nature of hydrocarbon detonations, *Proc. Am. Petroleum Inst.*, **39**, 15.

353. Pipkin, O. A. (1959) Detonation – old processes are not immune, *Proc. Am. Petroleum Inst.*, **39**, 21.

354. Strehlow, R. A. and Baker, W. E. (1975) The Characterisation and Evaluation of Accidental Explosions, NASA CR 134779.

355. Jacobs, R. B., Bulkley, W. L., Rhodes, A. B. and Speer, T. L. (1957) Destruction of a large refining unit by gaseous detonation, *Chem. Eng. Prog.*, **53**, 565.

356. Randall, P. N., Bland, I., Dudley, W. M. and Jacobs, R. B. (1957) Effects of gaseous detonations, *Chem. Eng. Prog.*, **53**, 574.

357. Pfreim, H. (1941) Reflexiongesetze fur ebene druckwellen großer schwingungsweite, *Forsch. Arb. Geb. Ing.*, **12**, 148 and 244.

358. Gerstein, M., Carlson, E. R. and Hill, F. U. (1954) Natural gas–air explosions at reduced pressures, detonation velocities and pressures, *Ind. Eng. Chem.*, **46**, 2558.

359. Luker, J. A. and Leibson, M. J. (1959) Dynamic loading of rupture discs with detonation waves, *J. Chem. Eng. Data*, **4**, 133.

360. Randall, P. N. and Ginsburgh, I. (1960) Bursting of tubular specimens by gaseous detonation, *ASME Trans. Paper No. 60-WA-12*.

361. De Malherbe, M. C., Wing, R. D., Laderman, A. J. and Oppenheim, A. K. (1966) Response of a cylindrical shell to internal blast loading, *J. Mech. Eng. Sci.*, **8**, 91.

362. Brossard, J. and Charpentier de Coysevox, M. (1976) Effets d'un confinement souple sur la detonation des mélanges gazeux, *Acta Astronautica*, **3**, 971.
363. Brossard, J. and Renard, J. (1981) Mechanical effects of gaseous detonations on a flexible confinement, 'Gasdynamics of Detonations and Explosions' (eds J. R. Bowen, N. Manson, A. K. Oppenheim and R. I. Soloukhin), *Prog. Astro. and Aero.*, **75**, 108.
364. Ross, C. A., Strickland, W. S. and Sierakowski, R. L. (1977) Response and failure of simple structural elements subjected to blast loadings, *Shock Vib. Dig.*, **9**, 15.
365. Gaydon, A. G. and Wolfhard, H. G. (1979) *Flames, Their Structure, Radiation and Temperature*', 4th edn, Chapman and Hall, London.
366. Burgoyne, J. H. and Williams-Leir, G. (1948) The influence of incombustible vapours on the limits of inflammability of gases and vapours in air, *Proc. Roy. Soc.*, **A193**, 525.
367. Vanpee, M. and Shirodkar, P. P. (1979) A Study of Flame Inhibition by Metal Compounds, *17th Symp. (Int.) Comb.*, Comb. Inst., Pittsburgh, p. 787.
368. Palmer, K. W. (1973) *Dust Explosions and Fires*, Chapman and Hall, London.
369. Field, P. (1982) *Dust Explosions*, Elsevier, Amsterdam.
370. Bartknecht, W. (1981) *Explosions, Causes, Prevention, Protection*, Springer-Verlag, Berlin.
371. Lask, G. and Wagner, H. G. (1963) Influence of Additives on the Velocity of Laminar Flames, *8th Symp. (Int.) Comb.*, Williams and Wilkins, Baltimore, p. 432.
372. Maisey, H. R. (1965) Gaseous and dust explosion venting, parts 1 and 2, *Chem. and Proc. Eng.*, **46**, 527 and 662.
373. National Fire Protection Association (1954) *USA Guide for Explosion Venting, National Fire Codes 9*.
374. Bradley, D. and Mitcheson, A. (1978) The venting of gaseous explosions in spherical vessels, parts 1 and 2, *Comb. and Flame*, **32**, 221 and 237.
375. Harris, G. F. P. and Briscoe, P. G. (1967) The venting of pentane vapour–air explosions in a large vessel, *Comb. and Flame*, **11**, 329.
376. Nettleton, M. A. (1975) Pressure as a function of time and distance in a vented vessel, *Comb. and Flame*, **24**, 65.
377. Nettleton, M. A. (1978) Some features influencing the venting of vessels in which pressure gradients initially exist, *Fire Prev. Sci. and Tech.*, No. **19**, 4.
378. Ministry of Labour (1965) Guide to the use of flame arresters and explosion reliefs, *Safety, Health and Welfare Series*, No. **34**, HMSO, London.
379. Nettleton, M. A. (1976) Venting explosions: an empirical approach, *Fire Prev. Sci. and Tech.*, No. **14**, 27.
380. Morton, V. M. and Nettleton, M. A. (1977) Pressures and their venting in spherically expanding flames, *Comb. and Flame*, **30**, 111.
381. Burgoyne, J. H. (1967) Designing for protection against dust explosions, *Chem. and Ind.*, 854.
382. Harris, R. J. (1983) *Investigation and Control of Gas Explosions in Building and Heating Plant*, E. and F. N. Spon, London.
383. Cybulski, W. (1965) *Selected Translations on Explosions*, Scientific Publications Foreign Cooperation Centre of the Central Institute for Scientific, Technical and Economic Information, Warsaw.

384. Lee, J. H. S., Ostrowski, P. P. and Wu, J. H. J. (1976) Shock attenuation by a single transverse slit, *J. Fluid Mech.*, **76**, 675.
385. Grumer, J. and Bruszak, A. E. (1971) Inhibition of coal dust–air flames, *USBM Report No. 7552.*
386. Egerton, A. C., Everett, A. J. and Moore, N. P. W. (1953) Sintered Metals as Flame Traps, *4th Symp. (Int.) Comb.*, Williams and Wilkins, Baltimore, p. 689.
387. Broshka, G. L. and Will, R. G. (1975) *A Study of Flame Arresters in Piping Systems*, Project 3721, Amoco Oil Co., Naperville, Illinois.
388. Terao, K. and Kobayashi, H. (1982) Experimental study on suppression of detonation waves, *Jap. J. App. Phys.*, **21**, 1577.

Author index

Subject index